Pregnancy Notes
Before, During & After

Pregnancy Notes
Before, During & After

Rujuta Diwekar

w

westland publications ltd

61, II Floor, Silverline Building, Alapakkam Main Road, Maduravoyal,
Chennai 600095
93, I Floor, Sham Lal Road, Daryaganj, New Delhi 110002

First published by westland publications ltd 2017

ISBN: 978-93-86224-89-7

Typeset by Ram Das Lal, New Delhi, NCR
Printed at Manipal Technologies Ltd, Manipal

Contents

A Personal Note

When someone recently commented on a picture of mine post a yoga class and said I looked fat, I realized how insensitive people can be even if a woman has just delivered.

It got me thinking about how women must feel about (and deal with) changes in their body post delivery. Maybe their world shatters, maybe they feel so under-confident that getting back into fab shape starts feeling like a faraway dream.

And so I prodded Rujuta to write a book, this time on pregnancy and how to stay healthy before, during and post it.

Rujuta has written a beautiful book. But before you

get around to reading it, I just want to share with you what I learned during my pregnancy and post-delivery, my personal notes you can call them:

1. Work on getting fit even before you get pregnant. Since 2007, I have made a conscious effort to eat correctly, exercise and generally lead a more disciplined life. When Rujuta and I started on this journey, marriage was not even on the cards, and pregnancy wasn't even a faint idea in my heart; it started with getting in shape for a role and evolved into a lifestyle.

    So, for you, if it starts with getting in shape for a wedding, job, holiday, choose your diet plan cautiously and ask yourself the big question — does it have the potential to evolve into a lifestyle? And if it cannot and is something that's just a two-day or a two-month affair, drop it. If I could shoot during pregnancy, walk the ramp and travel the world, it's only because my body was healthy. Healthy enough to do some heavy lifting and not feel tired just because I was pregnant. Getting back into shape post pregnancy was the work of my commitment to eating right for the last ten years. I look the way I do because I have been at it for a decade, and not because of what I did or didn't do in the last two weeks or immediately post my delivery.

2. Pregnancy is a physiological milestone, don't confuse it with a sickness — and surely don't let the people around you, including your doctor, treat it like one. Do you have to be careful of hydration, meal timings or calcium intake? Yes. But do you have to give up on living your life and make it all about the pregnancy and the growing stomach? No. And this is exactly why a history of staying healthy helps.

The one time when heaps of advice gets loaded on you is during pregnancy. Eat this, don't eat that. Don't drink this. Don't take up that role, etc. Emotionally also, it's the most vulnerable stage a woman can go through. It's the one time that you may actually consider every random advice coming your way and worse, implement it. A friend of mine went on doodhi juice, another stopped exercising, and we all know many who quit their careers due to their pregnancy. It's not the time to start or stop anything, it's the time to take everything in your stride, to go on. So keep up with eating wholesome food, don't let some random fool tell you that it has too much carbs or fat or whatever. Wear the clothes you want and don't limit yourself to mommy's section or whatever. You are alive, with another life inside you, so if anything, live every moment twice, don't fret, you are doing just fine.

3. Mother Nature has your back. Just like pregnancy gives you a specific shape, albeit a round one, post delivery too, you are in a specific shape. Don't be in a rush to get rid of it. The extra fat is required for many important tasks such as lactation and protection of both the baby and the mom from infections and illnesses. If you have been doing it right, have a long history of fitness and ate right through the pregnancy, then just like the body grew, it will also shrink back naturally. The key here is patience and compassion. Eating very little, or nothing, in a bid to lose that weight is just silly.

In that sense, I am really fortunate to be surrounded by women who truly care about me. I remember specifically the conversation between me and Rujuta post my delivery when I told her to put me on the Tashan diet. She said no, we have to be careful, compassionate, feed the body well or risk hormonal imbalances later. Lolo was in agreement with Rujuta. She had knocked off some 25 kgs post her second delivery and famously done it eating rice and fish curry, and she in my eyes is the fittest mom out there. And Saif, on his part, told me women are inherently beautiful so they really shouldn't bother with losing weight, it's the men who really need to get their act together. Very sweet he is, I know.

4. Don't forget yourself after you deliver. Give your body some recuperation time. Pregnancy is tough, delivery is tougher and the toughest job of your life, motherhood, is just about to start. It takes a village to raise a child, goes a famous African proverb. So surely allow your family to help you with the baby — the husband, maasi, older cousins, let them spend some time with the baby while you get some peace and time to yourself. Having your own life, staying healthy, keeping up with your worklife are all important for the baby. A baby who grows up around a healthy and happy mom can build a good life for herself and contribute towards society much more meaningfully. We even have science now

backing this up: sons of working mothers are kinder and daughters are smarter. Not having a life of our own doesn't automatically turn us into great mothers, nor does being skinny. So be kind to yourself.

Pregnancy and motherhood are fun, if you are ready to enjoy every change in the body, every milestone with your baby. Mother and child is a bond that transcends waistlines, religious lines, borders and beliefs. Here's to all of us, the women of today and the children of tomorrow.

Kareena Kapoor Khan
Mumbai
April 2017

1

Preparing for Pregnancy

THE BIG DEAL

Not very long ago, young married women would visit a gynaecologist to get advice on how to not get pregnant before they were ready. Now we visit them to know how to get pregnant before it's too late. Women, somehow, now more than ever, feel that they are on some kind of deadline, and that if they don't pop a baby now, it may be never.

The truth is that we are living longer and we are also getting fatter. All of us are, but more so the urban woman, the one with access to education but not playgrounds. With access to jobs, but no free or me time. The big DEAL — our Diet, Exercise, Activity and Lifestyle (alcohol, smoking, stress, sleep) is making us fatter than what our mothers were when they were our age, and more prone to this condition of diabesity. It is the marriage of diabetes and obesity, and we are getting there through the route of insulin resistance. We may not be exactly obese, but we sure feel heavy in our bodies. We may not exactly have diabetes, but we sure have painful or irregular periods, breakouts and that invincible sweet tooth. Essentially, all signs that we are not regulating our blood sugars as well as we ought to, and that our insulin sensitivity needs a bit of a push.

This push comes from making long-lasting improvements to your diet, exercise, activity and lifestyle. No shortcuts here; the plan has to be something that is long term, irreversible almost, because once the baby pops out, you can't push it up the vaginal canal. Grossed out? But it's a fact. The Upanishads say that food determines both the fertility and protection of progeny. And yet, amongst the things that we undervalue, is the role of food in our reproductive health. In fact, that's exactly why I decided to write this chapter.

> We obsess about what to eat once pregnant, or what we should do to lose weight post-pregnancy, but pay very little attention to food before we get pregnant — and that really is the game-changer.

Here's a breakdown of what you must do with your diet, exercise, activity and lifestyle to help you get pregnant and have a healthy pregnancy.

1. Diet

The thing is, without good food, your hormones cannot be in a state of balance. Your hormones decide your sex drive, fertility, and this in turn defines how easy pregnancy is going to be and how quickly you can knock off the weight you have gained. Essentially, eating right today can make it extremely easy for you to both get pregnant and get back in shape post it, but you must act now. Now can be anytime, but surely a year before you get pregnant.

And, as step one, ditch the obsession with losing weight. I know, I know, the advice you hear first when you visit your gyny is to lose weight as it is supposed to increase your chances of conception. Sorry, but that is not quite how it works. The only thing that improves your chances of conception other than good sex, is insulin sensitivity. And to improve insulin sensitivity and reduce insulin resistance, you will have to take the brave path of increasing your lean body weight. And what you eat plays a big role in that.

So here are the top **five diet tips** to improve insulin sensitivity and make getting pregnant easy:

1. *Reduce intake of packaged products.* Essentially, don't eat anything that has a nutrient label on the packet. Be it cereals, milk or just biscuits, no more packaged food for you. Especially the low-fat versions of yogurt, cheese or even ice cream. Similarly, stay away from sugar-free products, whether it's a cupcake, cola or simply a grain-free croissant (whatever that means). The thumb rule is that if it's selling on the basis of a single nutrient or ingredient — on the presence or absence of it — then stay away. E.g. gluten-free, low-fat, high-protein, etc. — if this is why you

are buying it, then you have fallen for a ploy that is milking profits off the current villain or hero of the weight-loss market, leaving you poorer in both your wallet and health. Btw, have you heard the latest? Gluten-free is now linked to Type 2 diabetes. So much for you believing that it is the cause of your thyroid, obesity and flatulence. Get real, take the effort to educate yourself on the basics of food.

2. *Eat according to the season.* Recently I published a document online (available for free download on my FB page and website), which lists the fruits, vegetables, grains and pulses that one must eat while they are in season. Today, with everything being available in the market all the time, the millennials have lost the wisdom of what to eat and what to avoid depending upon the season. Remember, you get everything year round because it's frozen in some large cold storage. So make that logistical move from mall to a small market and patronize the stuff that is in season. Other than tasting better, it will also improve your chances of eating a variety of fruits and vegetables throughout the year. Improved diet diversity is

good news for the intestinal mucosa, probiotic bacteria and insulin sensitivity.

3. *Introduce a pickle or chutney* in one of your main meals every day. These may not be taught to us as sources of Vit B12 in schools or even nutrition colleges, but it is exactly these essential fat-packed side dishes that help us assimilate and even make our own B12. You can choose from peanut, til, coconut chutney to mango, mirchi, mushroom pickle based on your taste buds and the region you live in. One tsp of pickle to breakfast or lunch, and two-three tsp of chutney to lunch or dinner provides the body with a dose of essential fats, herbs and spices that are cleverly mixed to improve insulin response. Besides making the meal interesting, it lowers the glycaemic index of the overall meal, thus allowing insulin to respond optimally. This optimization of insulin response could well be the reason why the body craves for pickle during pregnancy, at least that's what our Hindi movies teach us.

4. *Learn to set curd at home.* Better still, find a husband who can do it for you. From the diverse

strains of gut-friendly bacteria to the essential amino acids and B vitamins, dahi is the magical food that you can't afford to miss. The probiotic yogurt in the market is no match for home-set curd. The home-set curd is also a good antidote to breakouts and sweet cravings during PMS and it will help keep acidity under control once pregnant, especially during the first trimester. Have a bowl every day and have it with a meal for best results.

5. *Know when to stop eating.* Follow the Mental Meal Map (also available on my website and fb page). Act as if you are in a café where there is no Wi-Fi; well, that's the route all hi-fi cafés across the globe are going. They want people to spend time with themselves or have meaningful conversations and simply focus on the food that they are eating, while they are at the café. It invariably leads to people feeling satiated with half the portion of what they typically eat. Half price mein double mazaa. This is also the agenda of the Mental Meal Map, where you first visualize how much you want to eat and then start with half the amount. The trick is to eat it in double the

time you typically take. It means smaller morsels of food enter the stomach, thus improving the micronutrient assimilation and insulin response. This process can be repeated if required, but the key is to be without gadgets during meal times. This was one of Kareena's well-kept secrets (when she says she eats everything), till she shared it on our fb live chat.

This also allows for natural fluctuations in the appetite based on the season, the company you keep or simply the phase of the menstrual cycle you are in.

Also, I would like to believe that I don't need to say it, but don't forget those three to five tsp of ghee every day.

TALKING DIETS

Children of Men, a movie released in 2006, is set in 2027, when women have become infertile and it's been eighteen years since the last baby was born. And then, interestingly, a girl of African

---

origin gets pregnant and she has to be protected, as that's the key to human survival. The movie is science fiction and uses war, the refugee crisis, etc., as a backdrop. I watched this movie on a cold December night and couldn't help thinking that this fiction may not really be so much fiction after all. Look around: infertility clinics have come up in every gully nukkad, your newspaper has a full-page advert on blood tests, and one in every five girls in India has PCOD (I suspect the numbers are even higher).

Science fiction thrillers to the Upanishads, the message is the same: war, losing open spaces, forests and mangroves to so-called development projects is going to cost us not just economically but may eventually put human survival itself at risk. This change in use of land is changing the way we eat. It is getting tougher to procure nutrient-dense food that is economically priced; and packaged food that is poor in nourishment is getting cheaper and more accessible. The next time you are talking about diet, this is what you should be talking about, not carbs, protein and fat. That only makes you a victim of the weight loss, food and even the pharma industry. It sets you on the path of one diet after another, knocking off a few kilos only to allow them to creep back on your body, and trying one pill after another to regulate your period cycle.

With these basics of food in place, you are going to feel energetic enough to exercise. So that is going to be the next thing we discuss.

2. EXERCISE AND ACTIVITY

Activity

Activity often gets mixed up with exercise, but they are two different things, and doing one increases your propensity towards the other. You must have heard about truck drivers losing sperm mobility and fertility due to long hours of sitting and the heat that it generates in the genital area. All of us on our hot seats and cool gadgets are pretty much versions of that truck driver, complete with UTI and even the itch. What you need is to move more than what you are currently doing, stand often, take a little walk around your house or office; in fact, sit only if there's nothing else you can do about it. Sitting and the lack of physical activity (PA) it brings is now a well-documented and independent risk factor, just like smoking is. It means that if you generally eat right and work out, but just sit around too much, then it still leaves you vulnerable to cardio-metabolic diseases. Sitting is the new smoking. In fact, just fifteen minutes of activity per day reduces the risk of heart diseases. Fifteen minutes is very little, but exercise science studies point out that we aren't even moving that much.

Activity is like the little sister of exercise: if you stay active you are much more likely to exercise and vice versa. So sitting for less time and moving your body, your muscles, really is critical to good health, and the baby will inherit this health so don't be casual about physical activity and exercise.

Exercise

Exercise is doing PA in a structured manner and with much more intensity. E.g.: walk to the store to buy a yoga mat or onions — activity. Walking, interspersed with running repeated five times and for a total of thirty minutes — exercise. Get it? The reason why obesity, PCOD and thyroid are supposed to come in the way of you getting pregnant is because they come in the way of regulating your blood sugars properly. And exercise is the medicine for that, with the additional benefits of improved mood, sex drive and egg/sperm quality.

In pharmacology, there is something called a 'target-dose-response' relationship and that is exactly what plays itself out here too. The target is the muscle, the dose is exercise and the response is better blood glucose control. No exercise for ten days and the OGTT test will show almost double the amount of insulin. OGTT is the oral glucose tolerance test (or OGCT, oral glucose challenge test) that is often done on pregnant women to check their propensity for gestational diabetes. Just one bout of exercise and the insulin sensitivity comes back and continues to stay strong for the next seventy-two hours.

To put it simply, if you don't pack more muscle than what you currently have on your body, then you are jeopardizing everything: conceiving, having a healthy pregnancy and getting back in shape post-pregnancy.

> More muscle means reduced insulin resistance, it means better implantation of the foetus, less risk of gestational diabetes while pregnant, and accelerated fat-burning and recovery post-pregnancy.

To gain more muscle, you have to do many unconventional things — and we will go over them a step at a time. But for now, remember — unlearn 'lose weight' and learn 'gain muscle'.

Why is exercise discouraged? Most diets and weight loss programs discourage exercise, especially strength training as it actually hampers loss of body weight. Drastic reduction or extreme methods with food eat into existing muscle and bone tissue and lead to an instant drop in body weight. No exercise, or only brisk walks, add more fuel to the fire and ensure that the loss of muscle tissue is further accelerated. The result is quick weight loss in the short term and slowly creeping fat, along with insulin resistance, in the long term.

Why you should gain muscle. When you gain muscle, you don't load your weight-bearing joints like the back, knee, ankle; instead, you begin to feel lighter on your feet. You don't or may not lose weight, you may even gain some weight, but you feel like you've shrunk, your clothes fit differently and people begin to compliment you on your weight loss. Your sleep quality improves, your sex drive shoots up and you no longer need an app to tell you that you are ovulating. Your work productivity improves, so do your moods, and even your tolerance for bitchy colleagues. Basically, you feel like you are ready to do some heavy lifting. And that, ladies and gentlemen, is the first step towards motherhood. Doing more, expecting less.

How to gain muscle. I suspect you knew this was coming — strength train. Resistance training, or weight training as it's commonly called, is an excellent way to not just build stronger muscles and a tauter skin, but also to improve the strength of tendons, bones, ligaments and joints. Without the necessary stimuli of resistance training, our bones weaken and become porous much before we age. Do you know why pregnant women are put on calcium supplements? Because in the absence of adequate calcium, the foetus is evolutionarily primed to pick it from your bones instead.

Two things you must know here:

1. Without the stimuli of exercise on the weight-bearing joints, the body is least interested in absorbing calcium whether it comes from food or from a supplement.

2. Without adequate bone density, your pregnancy will be a tiresome affair, riddled with aches, pain and swelling.

So weight train and make gains both on muscle tissue and the bone mineral density to carry the baby for the full term without running out of energy and patience.

The other big factor is insulin resistance — yes, again. The more muscle you carry, the easier it is for the cells of the body to pick sugar (nutrients) from the bloodstream and this helps lower the blood sugar level. During pregnancy, the body will reduce the insulin sensitivity a bit to make more nutrients available for the foetus. This is a double-edged sword, and without adequate muscle tissue, your body will have a tough time adjusting to it. And that's exactly why a lot of women with no history of diabetes develop gestational diabetes during pregnancy. It's not really age that comes in your way, it's lack of fitness and that, my dear, is easily preventable.

More details in Notes on Exercise on page 174.

MALE FERTILITY

Whenever we are working with couples for diet and exercise modifications, they invariably get pregnant. This is because they learn to exercise, eat intelligently, be stress-free and understand the importance of leading a disciplined lifestyle. When I work just with the wife, I secretly hope that the husband signs up too. Because when I have both, the lifestyle changes come easily.

When two happy, healthy people have sex, babies naturally come their way. This fact has often caused embarrassing circumstances for my forty and above clients, including the ones who had made peace with their 'can't have babies' status or the ones whose first one came after years of struggle and IVF. The naturally conceived baby is a big confidence booster for them and an equally happy (predictable) moment for us.

It's not just the right nutrition but the fact that one is now much more insulin sensitive now; it actually reverses ageing, and makes the forty-year-old, thirty from within. What we have to remember is that while PCOD and thyroid and obesity of women are well documented hindrances in their fertility, their partners' stress levels, lethargy and obesity are bigger factors that almost go unnoticed. When the man is at ease, sex is not just fun but making babies is a piece of cake, that you can both have and eat.

3. LIFESTYLE

How well you lead your life, is lifestyle — don't confuse it with eating avocado, travelling first class or carrying an LV. It's really about leading a regulated, disciplined daily life. Are you cool enough to wake up, latest, two hours after sunrise and sleep before midnight? Party, but not daily? Choose your invites and don't load up plates because buffets need to be vasooloed? It's really about whether you are grown up in your head and heart. Are you capable of self-regulation and making educated choices with food, fitness and well-being, or are you still attending five-day weddings because food and booze are paid for and it makes for good Insta pics? So while the need of the hour is to have a complete relook on how you have been living till now, here are a few things that need your active attention.

Alcohol and smoking. Disturbs the hormonal environment, comes in the way of mineral absorption and increases risk to developing insulin resistance. So be cool about it and drop these habits if you are planning to conceive.

Chai and coffee. If you need one after lunch, on

waking up or simply to think or sit up straight, you are just too unfit to even carry your own body weight. So go back to basics — clean up your diet, commit to regular exercise and regulate your bedtime. Soon enough the dependency will drop, you will need much fewer cups to get through the day, up to two-three max, and none of them will make or break your routine life.

Stress and sleep. Interconnected and interdependent, these two are the critical pathways of getting and staying pregnant, and before that, just being plain healthy. Stress, whether it comes from a relationship, job or anything else is not worth having. Challenges are a good thing, but when you feel that getting through each day is like going to a war, it's time to step back and rethink the path you want to take in your life.

A stressed-out body and brain is unable to sleep. Poor sleep is the harbinger of hormonal imbalance, reducing your chances of good health, good sex and good babies. You should be tired enough to sleep and you should sleep enough to recover from that tiredness, ready to face the day feeling as fresh as a daisy.

A nap in the afternoon, often called beauty sleep, will go a long way in helping you de-stress and sleep better at night. But then, you can't overdo a good thing — the nap works best when it's under twenty minutes.

More details under Notes on Sleep on page 194.

POLLUTION

Some pollution we can control at our individual level, like smoking, but largely this is one factor that governments must take active part in. The recent spike in Delhi's pollution led to a 30 per cent decrease in people's sex drive. Essentially, anything that makes us sick also reduces our ability to conceive / reproduce. Like insulin resistance, air pollution, too, reduces our body's ability to pick nutrients from the bloodstream because the toxins interfere with nutrient assimilation. On the other hand, a very interesting study revealed that women who were in the first trimester of their pregnancy during the Beijing Olympics gave birth to babies that were heavier than the average size of

---

babies born in that city. This is due to the fact that the Chinese government had taken proactive steps to reduce pollution over Beijing in preparation for the Olympics. Interestingly, babies of women in their last trimester during the Olympics weren't bigger or healthier than the average. Clearly, conception and early pregnancy, where risk of miscarriage is high, respond positively to cleaner environments. So if you miscarry routinely or are in a healthy marriage but not conceiving, check if you live in a polluted area. Shift, make a baby, and return in the second trimester. Not a bad alternative to all the things we are willing to risk and try for a pregnancy.

2

Pregnancy Food Rules

Pregnancy is a natural physiological state of being. And as weird as it sounds, your body has been preparing for it right from the time that you were a teenager, in fact right after you turned eight. The reproductive system — the vagina, ovaries and uterus — grow and mature into a healthy state only if accompanied with the right mental preparation. And that's why, traditionally, the formal education of the shastras, the scriptures, begins at the age of seven, so that the mind is prepared to grow and reach maturity along with the body.

One of the things you study early on is the Taittreya

Upanishads, also called the education chapter. They are full of instructions on anna or food; where it comes from, what it does, when to eat, etc., and interestingly, these are presented as a dialogue between a father and his son. They also talk about the journey of anna to become the Annamaya Kosha or the physical body, its ability to increase prana or energy, to stabilize the mana, sharpen the intellect and help you find bliss and joy in daily life. The view of the scriptures is that education is incomplete without understanding all aspects of anna, and without it progeny cannot grow, success remains elusive, and life itself becomes a burden.

> So both the mind and the body are prepared for maturity through anna or the right food; more importantly, the right attitude towards it. Education without this understanding is considered incomplete.

Essentially, very different from today's system where we learn about food as carbs, protein, fat, calories, etc., in school, and over a period of time develop a complex about our own body instead of understanding it. We go through weirdness about breasts and periods during our teenage years, and confusion about career or life itself in our twenties. And then, when we get pregnant, we fuss even more about what is happening to us or is about to happen, what to eat, what to avoid, and how to go about life in general from here on. And the big question — will the body shape change forever?

No, it will not and it's only a matter of time before you fit right back into those skinny jeans and sport those washboard abs. And if you go by the Upanishads, eating right would be simple, broken into some really straightforward steps. And so we have these easy-to-understand and easy-to-follow rules that are built on the fundamentals of yogic wisdom and its marriage with modern nutrition science. They will answer all food-related doubts during pregnancy, ensure a smooth delivery, and prepare you to be in good shape post pregnancy. They will also help tackle the common risk factors of pregnancy: high blood sugar or lowered insulin sensitivity, acidity or bloating, BP or swollen feet, low energy or lethargy. We will then use these very rules to build on a trimester by trimester plan of what to eat and when.

If done the right way, these pregnancy food rules will:

(a) Keep total pregnancy weight gain in the range of 6 to 15 kgs.

(b) Ensure optimum delivery of nutrients to the foetus.

(c) Keep the hormones in a state of balance both during and post pregnancy.

(d) Ensure you lose most of the pregnancy weight on the delivery table, with the rest of it coming off, like on auto-pilot, within the next four to six months.

(e) Prepare you mentally and physically with the task of raising a child.

But before we discuss the rules in detail, it's important to get clarity on this crucial but overlooked aspect which plays a starring role in our health, especially during pregnancy — the gut bacteria.

THE PRE AND THE PRO-BIOTIC

Traditionally, the food that a pregnant woman must eat — dal-rice-ghee, raw banana, bhakri with chutneys, sabzis like doodhi, karela, pumpkin, etc. —

falls into the category that modern nutrition science now recognizes as pre-biotic. Prebiotics are foods for the probiotics: the friendly gut bacteria, the species that are necessary for our optimal health. Pregnancy and the hormonal flux that it brings disturb the gut environment and put you at a risk of what is called as dysbiosis. Dysbiosis is when one of the specie dominates, disturbing the diversity of the microbiota and putting you at risk of developing vaginal infections, food intolerances and even blunting your insulin response. During pregnancy, if you are on a progesterone pill, taking antacids, or living in a stressful environment, then you are at an even bigger risk. It also comes in the way of normal fat-burning processes and puts you at risk of getting heavier than what you would like to be.

Thankfully, the stuff that is good for you during pregnancy and protects your gut environment is easy-peasy, it's like goddess Annapoorna is smiling thoda extra at you nowadays. But it's not just you that she wants to feed — she also wants to feed the tiny little micro-organisms that live within you. Who would know better than her that when these micro-organisms are well fed, they keep checks and balances on the growth of harmful bacteria within you and allow diverse groups of friendly bacteria to not just survive but thrive. The relationship between you and this microbiome or microbiota (the entire community of these live micro-organisms within us) helps regulate the appetite, prevents constipation, vaginal infections, helps boost the immune system, produces vitamins like B12 and carries out multiple essential functions for the body.

It's easy to eat like this when you think in terms of regional, seasonal and genetically compliant recipes. One of the challenges of writing this book was to cater to the vast, diverse population that we are. Just dal-rice will have a thousand variants, so will dahi-rice; if at one place it is with tadka of til, then at another it is with aloo chokha. What you must remember is that all these are good combinations for the microbiome, ones that have the right combinations of resistant starches (RS) and short chain fatty acids (SCFA) to nurture, satiate not just the human host but the micro-organisms too. And all this long before the term prebiotic or probiotic was even coined. So do yourself a favour and relish this wisdom in its true essence. It's important to remember that English doesn't have a monopoly on science and that when your dadi speaks to you in her local lingo, there is science in there that nutrition labs are going to validate in the next fifteen-twenty years, if not earlier.

THE BESAN DOODH

It amazes me that this has been the preferred cleansing solution for babies and mommies alike. Such a clever combination of the prebiotic besan and probiotic milk! And since changes to the microbiome are also linked to pregnancy-specific discolouration of skin, pigmentation, cellulite and the like, this is such a non-toxic, chemical-free way to prevent that. Local solutions for global problems isi ko kehte hai.

Okay, so here we go:

PREGNANCY FOOD RULES

Eat food that

- Is easy to cook and digest
- Hydrates and works as a natural antacid
- Provides easy-to-assimilate amino acids
- Is rich in micronutrients like iron, folic acid, calcium

Rule 1 – Easy to Cook and Digest

This is probably the core of the food rules. Digestion slows down during pregnancy, and the process of cooking ensures that food is actually pre-digested even before you begin to chew it. And the whole point of eating is to get the rasa or the essence of food, the nutrients. It's these nutrients which, once assimilated well, will nurture you and be passed on to your baby to nurture her as well.

Cooking is an evolved art form, one that engages all your sensory perceptions, draws you within itself, and comes closest to a state of meditation. It's human creativity at its best and a reflection of true human nature, one that is caring, giving and sharing. Intelligent and insightful at the same time, this is one of the earliest human expressions of art. In terms of nutrition science, cooking of grains and vegetables helped remove the anti-nutrients from them, these are molecules like phytates and oxalates that exist naturally but come in the way of nutrient absorption. So no salads, no juices and chew on your fruit when it's ripe.

Also, fresh, local food and time-tested recipes are by default easy to cook and nutritious at the same time. The other reason why I say that it should be easy to cook is because I would like to see our children grow in a world where roles are not limited by gender. If it's easy, it's easier to get men to participate in and share the responsibility of cooking. Besides, if you have to cook it yourself, then it has to be an easy thing to do and not something that drains you even before you get to work or just the thought of which wears out your enthusiasm.

These food rules are not separate; they almost overlap into each other or are natural extensions of each other — the separation is only for logical understanding. The foods that are easy to cook and digest are also the ones that are hydrating in nature and keep acidity down. Let's now explore this aspect better.

Rule 2 – Hydrates and works as a natural antacid

What we eat plays a major role in maintaining hydration levels and also preventing acidity build-up. The water balance of the body is important through one's lifecycle, but that much more during pregnancy as the placenta and amniotic fluid depend on it. The total blood volume goes up and both thirst and urine secretion gets more frequent. The kidneys play a big role here.

Our kidneys are the silent workers of our pregnancy: they won't get the credit like the ovaries or uterus do, but without their proper functioning and fine-tuning, a healthy pregnancy is almost impossible. Through the trimesters they keep adjusting to the new 'normal' levels of fluids and electrolytes, and all that they ask is a little mindful eating from you to help them cope better. When supported with right eating and drinking, they ensure that BP and acidity levels are kept under check.

Here are a few ingredients that can tilt the balance in your favour when taken right, but can leave you dehydrated and, therefore, acidic or sick when consumed in excess amounts or in wrong proportions and combinations:

(a) *Sugar*: It's useful and helpful for the body in certain combinations but in high amounts will leave you feeling drained out. Also, the origin matters. Sugar from sugarcane is good, but that from corn (high fructose corn syrup) is not.

Sugar is like that fresh drop of water that falls from the sky: if it falls in muddy waters, it becomes muddy. Unfortunately, a lot of 'pregnancy foods' fall in that category. So sugar in biscuits, cookies, juices, cereals, flavoured milks and other such packaged 'health' drinks is like muddy water, don't have it. And when this same drop falls in your chai, it's fine, drink it. Or, for that matter, if it falls in your laddoo, kesar badam halwa or kheer.

Along with the origin, the quantity of sugar matters and decides whether what you are eating is healthy or just marketed as that. WHO and various other nutrition bodies, including diabetic associations, restrict the daily intake of sugar to six to nine teaspoons. Eating a predominantly local, regional diet, including laddoos, sherbets, etc., will never cross this limit. But just a glass of packaged juice or a bowl of cereal will, and it's important to remember that.

Quick checklist

Good sugar: Sugarcane and its derivatives, all seasonal fruits, neera, coconut water, homemade sherbets, homemade laddoos, barfis and halwa, sugar used as seasoning while cooking certain dishes, jaggery and ghee or jaggery and saunf post meals.

Bad sugar: Cakes, pastries, biscotti, biscuits, cookies, readymade sherbets and juices (tetrapacked or stylishly glass-packed), chocolates, brownies, ice creams, icing, readymade cereals of all kinds, protein biscuits, protein or other health powders that one mixes in milk (the ones with a typical profile of 9 gm protein, 28 gm carbs and 20 gm sugars per serving — that's four tsp in just one drink), cupcakes, etc.

THE DIVINE SUGARCANE

While most sugars keep terrible company, there are some that keep the company of the divine really. Sugarcane is one such source, long celebrated for its ability to increase fertility and sexual virility in India, it is now badnaam thanks to some random associations and name-calling. Sugar is the ghee of the 1970s. You all know the story, right? We were asked to avoid ghee because it was full of cholesterol and then, in 2015, cholesterol was hailed as a nutrient that is no longer of concern for overconsumption by the USDA. India, its doctors and dieticians should have known better, but when it comes to food, everyone is a fool. So ghee was out and markets opened for refined vegetable oil, rice bran oil and virgin olive oil.

Now history is repeating itself, sugar is out and sugar substitutes are coming in, so is stevia. Then finally by the time our daughters are pregnant, USA or the then superpower will make an announcement that sugar is actually therapeutic, the food of the yogis, the taste-enhancer, the fine-balancer, and then our daughters can denounce us more than ever. So to cut a long story short, sugar or no sugar, if you have packaged and processed stuff, then you are overloading the digestive system and more importantly, the kidneys. The dark chocolate, red velvet cake, biscotti, etc., are best left on the counter and sugar is best celebrated and used intelligently.

Sugarcane also has a cleansing and detoxifying effect on the entire body. It's especially useful when you are feeling super gassy or farting embarrassingly during conference calls or choosing to sit on cushioned chairs in restaurants to muffle the fart sound. The juice is good, so is jaggery, and even crystalline sugar, and depending on your trimester we are going to add these to your meals.

The other stuff that is really good and has natural sugars but different from sugarcane is neera, coconut water, milk. So are the sherbets that use therapeutic ingredients that keep the satsang of sugar — nimbu, kokum, khus khus. It's through these natural and fresh produce that the body feels better supported to keep acidity levels low and hydration levels high.

(b) *Salt*: Again, the namak in your nimbu pani will hydrate but most stuff that comes out of packets is a bad idea. So are options like popcorn while watching a movie or those chips that you are eating since you are 'allowed to gain weight now'. Like sugar, it is not salt itself but the company it is keeping which is going to make it a good or a bad boy. So anything over the counter is a big no, but a homemade bhaji or mathri or chivda will do the trick.

During pregnancy, the serum sodium levels actually fall as the blood volume goes up, and this could well be one of the reasons why women crave salty stuff. Earlier, they would mostly end up eating imli with some salt or pickle, both healthy and rich in nutrients and friendly bacteria enhancers. But now, as the palate has been trained to eat on the go and consume processed stuff, they mostly crave chips and chicken wings. If you have been eating junk, expect an exaggerated effect during pregnancy.

The unrefined or Himalayan or natural or coloured salt is especially good because it is not just sodium chloride but carries within itself multiple minerals and phytonutrients (which give it a particular taste, smell, colour and consistency) and other electrolytes too, like potassium and magnesium. These salts, often used in fasts, are great to keep the pH level of the body in place, beat bloating and prevent fluctuations in BP.

Quick checklist

Good salt: Pickle, papad, sherbet, khara singdana or the practice of putting kalanamak on fruits like guava, star fruit, amla, karvand, etc. Regular use of salt in cooking, salt in bathing water, the occasional pakora or wada made at home.

Bad salt: Packaged and processed biscuits, chips (ya, even your vegan, kale chips), packaged salted nuts and chakna items, processed cheese, butter, outside stuff like Chinese take-away, samosa, pizza, popcorn, burgers, etc., basically anything that is sold in a franchise model in malls and on highways.

A NOTE ON SALT

The USDA reversed guidelines on cholesterol in April 2015; the next one that is likely to get revised is on salt in 2020. Till now it was acceptable that salt should be minimized or avoided, just like what we thought of cholesterol. But research now shows that very low consumption of salt is linked to insulin resistance, ageing and even heart disease. The USDA also came up with something called 'voluntary sodium targets' for food companies and restaurants, because more than 75 per cent of sodium that Americans eat comes from packaged, processed and restaurant foods, and not as namak in their nimbu pani or sabzi. Salt restriction needs to be understood as a surrogate measure of restriction on eating out, eating out of packets, etc., and not on mathris, papads, pickle and other nutritious foods made at home.

(c) *Caffeine*: The cup or two of chai or coffee with sugar will not harm, but caffeine crawls up from many unseen places — chocolates, cupcakes, energy drinks and colas — and it's through these things that it will leave you dehydrated.

So while you don't need to kick the cuppa, you must follow the basics:

1. No chai or coffee first thing in the morning, start with a fruit or dry fruit.

2. No chai or coffee as a replacement to a meal. E.g. in office during / after long meetings.

3. No chai or coffee as a late-night meal post dinner like when you step out to meet friends / go for a drive, etc.

All the above are applicable also to green tea or white tea or any other tea.

Basically, the thing to keep an eye on is your urine: if it smells of tea, coffee, you are overdoing it and need to cut back; especially the invisible sources as mentioned earlier.

And one more special pregnancy tip is to never have tea or coffee just before stepping out of the house. During pregnancy, the body maintains a delicate balance between its anti-diuretic hormone, hydration level and blood pressure, and a cuppa for the road may well leave you needing a loo, which in India you are not going to find easily. The best drink that will get you from point A to point B while keeping you hydrated without you needing to pee is a glass of milk.

(d) *Fibre*: Again, let it come from fruits, veggies, legumes and grains, but stay away from fibre drinks and pills. Because, in excess amounts, it can actually leave you both dehydrated and constipated besides coming in the way of nutrient absorption.

So watch out for the salads, soups, juices you might be drowning yourself in, in the name of 'fibre'. Eat real food, cook it well, allow your teeth to chew. Other than keeping your oral environment healthy, it will also lead to better secretion of digestive juices and prevent all the digestive disorders of nausea, constipation, bloating. A lot of antacids come with fibre too, so avoid those. Actually avoid all kinds of antacids because if you pay attention to following the food rules, acidity will be well within control. A little known fact about antacids is that they interfere with the absorption of nutrients like B12 and Vit D and you don't want to be falling short of that now.

Rule 3 – Provides Easy-to-Assimilate Amino Acids

Do you need more protein when you are pregnant? Yes, to support the growth of the foetus and for your own body's needs. But the only way your body will have access to more protein is if it comes in the form of easy-to-assimilate amino acids. These come from wholesome food; food that is rich in common sense, wisdom and passes the test of time.

The minute you get pregnant, one of the things that you are likely to hear from your gyny is that you must now increase your protein intake. But when we hear this, we are pretty clueless about exactly what to eat and what to avoid. Vegetarians wonder if they must now include eggs, others consider supplementing their diet with the many varieties of protein shakes that carry pregnant women on their packaging. But the truth, as always, lies somewhere in between. And that's why, again, the gold standard in food advice is to not take nutrient-based advice but food pattern -based, or more specifically, regional food pattern- based advice.

Our body goes through what is called daily protein turnover, where proteins are built and broken. Typically, on a day-to-day basis, this won't have an ill effect on your health, but if you are ageing, recovering from an injury or are pregnant (and not eating correctly), you will lose more protein than you build per day. This leads to hair loss, nail breakage and long-term losses of bone and muscle tissue, decreasing not just the total strength in your body but your actual functional capacity. That means that the heart, lungs, insulin begin to function at less than optimum rates, leaving you tired, fat and even diabetic. This is another reason why you will also see some women with no history of diabetes develop gestational diabetes.

For the body to not waste or eat into your existing muscle protein stores, you will have to plan your protein intake carefully. Gone are the days where you could do things like cereal for breakfast and protein for dinner. You have to eat in a way that improves protein assimilation post a meal (in technical terms — post-prandial protein synthesis) or risk complications with the foetal growth and loss of your muscle tone and bone density.

Along with amino acids in foods, the other nutrients that improve protein synthesis are essential fats, like those found in dairy and dairy products, minerals like those found in nuts, and phytonutrients, like the ones found in vegetables. It's really about distributing your protein intake through the day and consuming it as part of a nutrient-rich meal versus just ingesting protein on its own. A pre-sleep protein drink that is also rich in fat can further amplify protein synthesis and that's why it was common practice to feed an expecting mother a cup of milk as a bedtime snack. All this is incorporated in the meal plans for each trimester in the next chapter.

The muscle protein synthesis is also one of the main reasons why fasting or staying hungry for a long time during pregnancy is a bad idea as it leads to protein losses.

THE ESSENTIAL LEUCINE

The amino acid leucine is probably the most important amino acid during pregnancy as just the act of eating leucine improves protein synthesis and prevents muscle loss. Leucine belongs to a category of essential amino acids called branched chain amino acids (BCAA), which play an important role in hormone signalling and, therefore, assumes an important role before and right after delivery. And like love, leucine is found in places you may not be looking for: rice, nuts, legumes and dals, and then of course the usual suspects — milk and milk products, eggs, fish and meat (and, therefore, the importance of eating wholesome). Leucine improves insulin response, helps you lower blood glucose levels, reduces serotonin and, therefore, lowers the feelings of drowsiness and fatigue that are common during this time.

Rule 4 – Naturally Rich in Micronutrients

Micronutrients like folic acid, calcium and iron we all know of, but a healthy pregnancy needs an array of micronutrients, from the phyto-sterols to lycopenes, the flavonoids to the phyto-estrogens and the resveratrol to anthocyanins.

The foods rich in these micronutrients that really do the trick and leave you glowing, energetic and happy are the forgotten foods of India. The local, or shall I say, the hyper local, the stuff that doesn't have a name in English or even Hindi for that matter. The nawrangi dal of the high Himalaya, the jackfruit jam of Kerala, the cherry pickle of the North-East, the tender cashews of the Konkan coast, the smart use of the hemp seed in the east of India.

It's in these forgotten foods that you find a bank of nutrients that work as the agents that keep the body's acidity levels down and the blood sugar levels under check, and improve the health of the microbiome. These come into our diet through almost a secret route — the pickle, the chutney, the laddoo. And if you are going by conventional information on diet, you are most likely to miss out on them. Let's look at how.

- You may be told to consume more iron or folic acid and you must just rely on pills or drown yourself in a bowl of spinach every day without realizing that a handful of cashews or an aliv (garden cress) laddoo will load you on both the folate and the iron and that too without constipating you.

- Or you may avoid pickle because you fear that it has 'too much salt' and then land up missing out on many essential nutrients from the pickle, especially Vit K2. You may have never heard of Vit K2, or you may be completely unaware of its role in preventing bone loss and osteoporosis, but that doesn't mean that you won't benefit from it. One of my clients from Pune received a tiny bottle of amla achaar from her maternal grandmother on getting pregnant. This achaar was made by the grandmother's mother and kept solely for the use of pregnant girls in the household to protect their spines.

- Or you could be loading up on high-fibre packaged cereals or oats because you've been told it's healthier, little knowing that the phytate from it is going to block the absorption of many minerals in your body, more importantly that of magnesium. And then what we often overlook, but our grandmoms didn't, is that Vit K2 and magnesium are critical for Vit D absorption. Isn't that interesting in our world of Vit D deficiencies? And that together, these three protect the bones and even have a heart-protective effect.

To summarize — the pregnancy food rules help us make the right food choices and simplify the dizzyingly complicated world of pregnancy foods and nutrition for the mother and the foetus. They tell us that the 'dal-chawal-achaar' or 'khichdi-pickle-curd' meals are complete for the body and most of their real benefits are hidden and unknown. And that beyond carbs and calories lies a magical world full of heritage recipes, super foods and secret ingredients, whose custodians are our grandmothers and where healthy pregnancies are a norm. Let's explore this in the next chapter.

THE DATE AND THE BABY

On my flight back to Mumbai from London, I got upgraded to first class, but the best part was

---

yet to come. I put on my headphones and tuned into qawwalis in their music section. I stretched myself on the large seat, as big (or small based on perspective) as my bathroom, closed my eyes, opened my ears and tapped my feet to *Dama dam mast kalandar*. It was some local rendition, not by any known singer, and then, in one of the verses, there is a dialogue between the two qawwals, and they are telling the story of two sisters married for last fourteen years but both still without a child. Their sadness knows no bounds and then they hear of a fakir who has a 100 per cent success rate with infertility issues. The fakir gives them a date each and says, just eat this date in the morning and get on with your normal lives. One of the sisters eats the date, the other one doesn't. Lo and behold, nine months later, the sister who ate the date goes to visit the fakir with her little one in her arms. But he is shocked that the other sister is there without a baby. 'Did you not eat the date,' he asks her. 'No,' she says sheepishly. 'Do you remember where you put it?' 'Yes, by a rock on the hill.' 'Arre pagli, toh jaa, your child is waiting there for you.' The sisters run to the rock on the hill and find a little baby, right where she had put that date, kicking his legs up in the air and crying.

They say that from the times of the *Mahabharata*, every truth is fictionalized and presented like a story so that the listener may get the message in an easily digestible way. This story reaffirmed my belief that you don't just need shraddha and sex — without good food, babies won't come our way.

Special Note: Pregnancy and the Upanishads

According to yogic philosophy, we are all made of five elements or pancha mahabhoota, and these five elements follow an order: first comes space; from space, air; then fire; then water; and finally the earth. On earth there are various ooshadhi (medicine or herbs, for the lack of an exact translation) and from this comes anna or food.

- A baby is conceived within the space that exists inside the mother, and space has the quality of sound. So mothers can hear their baby within weeks of the pregnancy, quiet and otherwise submissive women begin to find a voice, and that strength, they will tell you, comes from the baby. And with ultrasounds these days, you will hear the heartbeat by the sixth week, long before the baby has taken any shape.

- Then comes the air element, and most women experience some disturbance within their body's vata or air element and will experience some degree of nausea or feel bloated or have a disturbed digestion.

- Then the fire element comes in and it has the quality of form, so over a period of time, the baby takes shape within the body and you can almost see her tiny feet and even nails in the ultrasound scan.

- Then eventually the water breaks and a baby — with the quality of earth, of being solid or immovable — is born. You can now hear, touch, see, taste and smell your baby and the first thing she will do on taking birth is seek the ooshadhi, the breast milk, and thanks to this first food, the baby will feel nurtured and eventually grow and mature into a fine human being.

We must eat in tune with these five elements, especially when nurturing a life within. Here is how:

Space: Take the time to hear your inner cues while eating. To do that you will have to learn to take the time to eat in a way where you are able to cut down on unwanted noise. So slow down your pace, find your space and eat.

- Do: Consciously assign meal times to yourself, at least the main meals of breakfast, lunch and dinner.

- Don't: Grab lunches, rush your meals or eat while watching TV programs.

Air: Eat your meals to a point of feeling light. This borrows from the first principle of space. When you slow down the pace at which you eat, you learn to eat to a point of lightness. When meals are rushed, people often feel that the food is all the way up to their throat, sometimes even the nose ;). So pay attention to feeling food going down your stomach and stop before it's full.

- Do: Use the Mental Meal Map and serve yourself smaller portions at one time.

- Don't: Practise portion control; instead focus on eating just right and have the flexibility to adjust portions based on your appetite at each meal.

Fire: Amongst the holiest elements, Agni is even worshipped as god, so eat food that is cooked or, as they say, purified by fire. So no re-heating of food in microwaves or opening packets of ready-to-eat meals. Eat home-cooked food and let it be cooked slowly on fire. The practice of feeding pregnant women first also comes from this, as the fire element of warmth is active in food when it is eaten fresh off the pan / stove.

- Do: Eat freshly-cooked food and consume within three hours of cooking. Make intelligent use of spices.

- Don't: Reheat food using microwaves. Don't eat vegetable salads or soups; while one is not cooked at all, the other is overheated. Balance is the key here.

Water: Keep the hydrating element alive in your food. This comes from water itself and eating fresh food. Stale food often feels drier than fresh food, so does eating out because of the lack of the hydrating element. Eating anything that's too sweet, or overdosing on tea, coffee, or colas, will also have a dehydrating effect on meals, so learn to strike that balance and, as Swami Sivananda says, avoid food that is old and cold.

- Do: Stay well hydrated and check that urine is clear at all times. Eat fresh fruit, drink local sherbets, nariyal pani, neera, etc. once a day.

- Don't: Overdose on tea / coffee. Especially quit the cuppa on rising, the dessert post lunch, and the midnight raid on the fridge for ice cream / chocolates.

Earth: This is pretty basic but is often overlooked due to all the diet fads around. Eat stuff that belongs to the region you are living in. Definitely all the fruits and veggies from your land, so banana and not the kiwi; poha, not the cereal. The less the food travels to land on your plate, the stronger you will be, and pregnancy is a test of strength in more ways than one. So sit down to eat, sit as close to the earth as you can, and eat what comes from the farms and not malls.

- Do: Fix a place to have meals and assume the cross-legged position to use gravity to your benefit. Also helps improve hip flexibility and digestion. Eat what is in season and stay rooted to your genetic preferences for meals.

- Don't: Consume ready-to-eat packets / meals, eat fruits and veggies that are out of season, e.g. — greens during the rains or apples in summer.

Now, of course, all this may seem too esoteric or very generic but it easily marries with what nutrition science has to say about the needs of pregnant women and the growing foetus.

3

The Three Trimesters

For each trimester:

- FAQs
- Top three foods
- Meal plan
- Important notes
- Heritage recipes

THE FIRST TRIMESTER (T1)

'I could smell the grease on the lift door, the coffee in the pantry even before I entered the office, and the nauseating smell of the deo my colleague was wearing. Something was odd today, everything smelled, even the traffic on the street, and that little plastic over the branding of my new Michael Kors.

'Shit, Google said heightened olfactory sense could be an early sign of pregnancy. I wanted to run out of my office, out on the streets where there would be no bathrooms and no scope to use a pregnancy kit. I didn't want to jinx it but I couldn't wait until the next morning either. "Just do it, Deepti," said a voice inside my head, and so did Jyoti from my team. "You know, you are if you are and you are not if you are not, no one is half pregnant." So, I went to the office loo, carrying my handbag with me. I could already smell the citrus bathroom freshener as I sat on the pot, held the kit under my vagina and forced myself to pee. Nothing. Nothing flowed. "Come on," I coaxed myself, just a couple of drops, and there, I got two. Two drops and two bars on that test. It was positive. Should have been the happiest moment, but it was probably the most cautious moment in all my thirty-six years of life.

'I walked out of the bathroom clutching the test kit in my hand, and at the sight of Jyoti, held it up for her to see. This woman Jyoti, who I half-hated, quarter-respected and quarter-loved was now the only person other than me who knew what was going on and I hated that. So I WhatsApped a pic of the test kit to my husband. Two blue ticks later, he replied, "Babe, these things could be wrong and you must talk to your doctor and set up an appointment for a blood test tomorrow." Wow! Everything about getting pregnant was like suhaag raat — it doesn't live up to its promise and almost no one knows how to respond to it at first.

'The questions were already floating in my head, though I should have waited until the blood test. So I took out a notepad and wrote down everything I wanted to know.'

So here goes:
FAQs for T1

1. Can I take the rickshaw back home or is it risky for the early foetus?

Darling, you can even take the parachute home. Hormonally, you are changing, priming actually, and unless you have been specifically asked to be on bed rest, you are good to go in a rickshaw. Pregnancy is the one time when the body's endurance abilities jump almost to an unnatural level, giving pregnant women an edge over non-pregnant women. This was a big scandal in the 1980s and the USA Olympic Committee even has a ban on what is called 'abortion doping'. It's the practice where female athletes get pregnant just before the games to exploit the physiological advantages that come with it. The increase in the red blood cells levels of the body, for example. The oxygen-carrying red blood cells not only improve nutrient delivery to the foetus but also increase the body's aerobic performance. Add to that the naturally high levels of the human growth hormone, progesterone, oestrogen and even relaxin that may give a further boost to your gymnastic or even power sport performance.

So, on the one hand, pregnancy is being treated like a performance-enhancing drug, and on the other, pregnant women are paranoid about lifting even their handkerchief from the floor in the fear of a miscarriage. At the Facebook Live that Kareena and I hosted, she went on record to say that women must not treat pregnancy like a disease. It's a natural physiological state and you can do everything you have been doing in your life and even more, like winning Olympic medals ;).

> The key here is to understand that, essentially, pregnancy will only amplify the state your body was in before you got there. So if you were healthy and fit, expect an amplification again.

If you were diseased and depressed, well, expect an amplification. Thankfully, there is no rush to get pregnant today; we are living longer than ever and have access to more resources than women had, say, just twenty years ago. So take my advice, get healthy before you get pregnant, and then you can glow like Kareena and do your version of walking ramps, shooting and looking like million dollars. And yes, take the rickshaw.

And while we are talking physiology, here's some psychology. If your relationship with your husband and in-laws was bad, then that gets amplified too. And if he's a good husband, then, well, some more goodness is coming your way. So in effect, pregnancy doesn't stand in your way nor does it make anything go away — it just makes everything bigger in your life.

P.S.: Serena Williams just won the Australian Open grand slam in her first trimester.

2. Should I stop exercising or start it?

Neither actually; just keep at what you are doing and, as usual, follow the thumb rule of exercise — listen to your body and take it easy when you need to. If you are a regular workout person (by regular I mean ten-fifteen years of consistent exercise), you will notice a big jump in your strength, flexibility and stamina levels. Workouts will be more fun than before. And since you are familiar with what you are doing, just keep up with your regular workout routine. So if you run, run; if you lift weights, lift weights; if you ski, ski. Your baby is lucky to be with you, and what better than to work out from the minute she is conceived.

However, if you are the kind that only took to exercise recently as a means to lose weight or on a doctor's advice and has more skipped sessions than done, well you need to take it easy. The first trimester is surely not the time to work out with a vengeance. If you were doing a day or two of exercise per week, just keep at it and reduce your intensity. This means, cut down on the speed and duration of your cardio exercises, reduce the numbers of sets, weights and reps on your weight-training exercises, and if you go to a group class, inform your teacher about your pregnancy. Cycling and swimming, the non-weight-bearing exercises, are better than walking, machines are better than free weights, and it's important that exercise is stopped before exhaustion hits in. Stay well hydrated during your exercise and wrap up your session with a banana. It's important to refuel immediately post exercise to help the body with its recovery processes.

And if you have never exercised, kya bolu, congratulations on the pregnancy and you can walk around as a means of activity, but don't start with any new form of exercise in the first trimester.

3. How much protein do I need now?

This is amongst our biggest confusion, protein and where to get it from, especially if you are a vegetarian. At the recently concluded sports and exercise conference in Newcastle, UK, there was a session on what was called 'The Kardarshian Index'. It's a scientific paper that talks about how scientific facts get lost or trivialized when sensationalized, and measures a scientist's social media following vis-à-vis the number of citations and peer review articles.

In the age of social media, it's not uncommon for someone to sound very scientific on food and nutrition but not really have any solid background in the field. A good quote and a good picture matters more than the truth. So things we have never heard of before come into our world as sources of protein — quinoa, chia and the works. And with that, the confusion of what you must eat to get more protein.

For starters, do pregnant women need more protein? Yes. Do you get a certain nutrient only from one specific food? Hell, no. We must eat food and not nutrients; food delivers much more than a single nutrient or multiple nutrients. Think of food as sex and a nutrient as a baby. Can sex lead to a baby? Yes. Is that the whole point of it? No. Without sex, life would lose its meaning, pushing the body into a state of hormonal imbalance and the mind into depression. Read that again if you need to.

And don't pick what to eat based on your understanding of whether it has protein, carbs or fat, because there is a good chance that your understanding may be far removed from scientific facts. And nutrition science has already moved to choosing meals based on food systems and not food groups, but the Kardarshian Index may have prevented you from being aware of this.

'More protein' is the sensational part of the scientific

fact of 'positive nitrogen balance'. To achieve a positive nitrogen balance you must not be on a calorie-restricted diet, should sleep on time and lead an active life. Now this is not something that you can fit into 140 characters, or you may not have the patience for it — and a wholesome approach is a tough one to sell. It's easier to just say — eat an egg every day, drink a glass of milk, include protein-rich foods in your diet. Because no one cares about the fact that without wholesome meals, sleep and exercise, the amino acids from these foods won't help you get into that positive nitrogen balance. And without nitrogen to spare, the foetus growth is seriously compromised. We have become people who believe that consumption is the same as assimilation.

Eating protein is not the same as *getting* protein, and surely not the same as getting protein to do its work of growing and protecting the foetus. Especially during pregnancy, as this is one time that the body's acidity levels are high due to higher progesterone levels, and digestion processes are behaving erratically.

One of the things that matters most with protein is its digestibility ratio, and a thumb rule to increase that is to eat protein-rich foods as a part of a complete meal and not on its own. So back to eating everything — actually, the word for it is eating intelligently, i.e., going beyond the superficial information on labels and tabloids.

4. Are there any special vitamins that I need to take?

The supplement industry would love for us to believe that there is one formula for hair and nails, another for kidney dialysis, and a special one for pregnancy. Vitamin marketing is a bit like cola marketing, it's the same cola that they have been selling you for ages, but they package it in different styles, bottles and sizes so that you feel that the one in your hand is really cool, yo! The difference, I must admit, is that while any cola of any size or packaging will take away nutrient assimilation from the food, the vitamins will only add to it.

The vitamins you need are the exact same that are required for the good health of women during the reproductive age — Vit D, calcium, iron, Vit B, with emphasis on folic acid (B9) and B12. If you have the budget for it, taking that special packaging wala vitamin is not gonna hurt, but if you are already a regular supplement user, then simply continue with your existing ones.

And you must remember that a supplement is just that, a supplement, not a replacement to eating right, exercising, sleeping on time and generally having a positive attitude towards life.

5. Why am I getting so sick every morning?

In part it is natural because of the changes in the hormonal status in the body. The high progesterone and growth hormones make it difficult for the body to keep the acidity down, but your eating habits can make it worse, or better, for you. So a lot of times it's not just the hormones but actually the lifestyle that leads to really bad nausea. Pay special attention to getting a good rest in the night: keeping gadgets away at least sixty minutes before bedtime is helpful for the hormones and allows the body to unwind. So is getting a quick nap of fifteen-twenty minutes every afternoon, right after lunch. Lastly, and very importantly, please just stop eating packaged stuff or take-outs.

6. Is there a special way to avoid nausea / morning sickness?

Yes, there is.

(a) Wake up to a fruit / dry fruit and don't have tea for the first two hours after rising.

(b) Add an extra dollop of ghee to lunch and dinner so that the blood sugars climb slowly and stay steady for a long time.

(c) Drink a glass of kokum sherbet with a pinch of kalanamak before noon as a midmorning meal.

(d) Have a warm water bath. Add freshly-cut lemongrass to your warm water — it has a relaxing effect on the body and mind.

(e) Right after your bath, take a tiny drop of coconut oil or ghee on your little finger and massage the insides of your ears with it.

7. Do I need more folic acid now?

You need food that is richer in nutrients and folic acid

counts too. The key here is to not entirely depend on the supplement but use it as an aid to support folic acid intake from natural foods. Beetroot, seasonal vegetables and an under-valued source is cooked lentils — moong, matki, chawli and the likes. Vit B12 is required for Vit B9 (folic acid) to carry out its functions, so don't forget the dahi, chaas, and again the soaked, sprouted and well-cooked lentils. The thing to remember is that nutrients depend on each other to carry out their specific functions. It's like your production department needs a well-functioning admin or maintenance department for it to work at its optimum.

There are some reports of excess folic acid doing more damage than good to the baby, but my guess is that is much more likely to happen if the diet is overall poor in nature and one is just popping a folic acid pill.

8. What to do about itchy nipples and navel?

This isn't unusual but can be unusually embarrassing because, you know, as girls we don't scratch just because it is itching, we leave that for the boys. The itchiness is due to the change in the hormones but gets out of control or causes redness, bruises, etc. only when accompanied with dryness that comes with a poor nutritional status. The way out is pretty simple:

- Massage your body with cold pressed til or coconut oil before a bath and avoid any fragrant soaps, oils or creams, as the chemicals will further irritate the skin.

- Take Vit E with dinner two to four times a week; ensure that your Vit D levels are up to the mark. Taking a supplement of 1000IU with lunch helps.

- Have soaked badam or nuts as a mid-meal once a day — the phyto-sterols and essential fats will run to your rescue. The other secret agents being your til /peanut / coconut or sunflower seed chutneys.

- Yoga is especially helpful since it regulates hormones and helps nurture both the skin and the digestive system, especially the inversions.

- And, of course, eat better, wholesome and on time.

A NOTE ON APPETITE

The one thing that pregnancy will give you is a larger blood volume, with the amniotic fluid and all. This change in your water balance in turn changes your appetite, which then influences how much you eat. And it's how much you eat that nurtures the body, enhances blood volume, and ensures that the amniotic fluid stays in a healthy state. Season, time of day, the daily stresses — all further influence your appetite. While you don't need to eat for two, or three for that matter, what you need is a compassionate view towards your appetite. Sometimes you are going to feel not very hungry, at other times mad hungry; at both extremes and in the middle, know that this is perfectly normal behaviour for a pregnant woman. Following a sensible routine and a disciplined lifestyle will ensure that the variation in the appetite stays in the healthy range and doesn't need medical attention. (The moon represents the water element in our body and if you follow the moon closely, you would notice a fluctuation in your appetite based on its size.)

The Top Three foods for T1

While writing this book, I figured that there is now an infobesity (overload of information) on every trimester: the hormones, the foetus, nutrients needed and everything. In spite of this, info on what to eat in terms of the Indian context is non-existent. And though the hormones and foetal growth will follow a universal pattern, the food part needs to be localized. The lost wisdom needs to be unearthed from our kitchens, translated from vernacular to a language that resonates with nutrition science, and more importantly, allow it to support the working woman both nutritionally and emotionally in this phase.

So, in every trimester, I am going to list out the three most important foods that you must incorporate in your plan and follow it with a recommended meal plan. Feel free to tweak the recommended meal plan based on your daily routine, but ensure that these three foods are not forgotten in the daily bhagdod of your zindagi.

The first trimester is easily the most challenging and critical part of your pregnancy, and though the baby will grow on auto-pilot from here on, there are some foods which will help you tide over this phase smoothly.

T1F1: Hing or Asafoetida

A common Indian herb or spice that has anti-bacterial, anti-viral properties and is a digestive aid. It's the one spice that will help keep the nausea and bloating down, stoke your appetite and help you eat better. Most of us use it in tadkas, especially for dals, and it aids absorption of nutrients from the dal. It also plays an important role in helping to improve our moods, and relieves fatigue or drowsiness that sometimes accompanies T1.

How to use it:

- Pinch of hing in chaas (buttermilk) along with kalanamak to keep the acidity down.
- In tadkas for dals and sabzis.
- Add a pinch in coconut oil and massage on the tummy for relief from gas and bloating.

T1F2: *Ragi / Nachni / Mandua or the Finger Millet*

India is the highest producer of this millet but affluent urban folk are almost unaware of this red little wonder. Or at least that was the case till the gluten-free fad struck us too. Ragi is a nutrient-rich food and — from amino acids to calcium, iron to fibre — it provides us everything that we need in this crucial phase. It regulates our appetite and prevents over-eating, is very easy to both cook and digest, and even keeps the lipid levels (triglycerides — the circulating fat in the bloodstream, high levels of which will make you prone to diabetes) in check. Also, long term it is required for good lactation too, so it's good to start including it in your meals, at least a couple of days a week, from now.

How to use it:

- Can make bhakris or rotis with it, and while this takes some practice, the ragi dosa is easy to make and delicious. Just dosa and chutney also makes for a light meal when you are not feeling like eating a full meal of roti-sabzi-dal. Ragi mudde, eaten with peanut chutney in Karnataka, is a good light meal too.

- Sprouted ragi is even better and can be stored / refrigerated for a week. Can turn into a quick breakfast meal — malt / satva or kanji or ambil — and you can teach your husband to cook this.

- Ragi laddoo, made by rolling it with sesame, almonds, peanuts and coconut. You can Insta it with the following hashtags: #glutenfree #miracleseeds #calciumrich #yummy #easytocook #dairyfreecalicum

T1F3: Beet

It's rich in the phytonutrient betalains, known for its antioxidant, detoxification and anti-inflammatory properties. And though beetroot is not a good source of iron (the leaves are), it's an excellent source of folic acid. It also contains high amounts of manganese, magnesium and copper, and even vitamins like B6 and C. This nutrition profile is good for nerve support, prevents calf pain and varicose veins too. If you can get your hands on beet leaves, eat them too by cooking them like a palak or spinach bhaji; it's a good source of iron and other minerals.

How to use it:

- Simply pressure or steam-cook it and eat a beetroot as a part of a meal or a mid-meal by itself.

- Beet poriyal is an excellent and nutrient-rich sabzi that's easy to cook.

- Add pieces of beetroot to rice or khichdi — easiest way to cook and eat.

The T1 Meal Plan

Timing	Meals	Notes
Meal 1 – On rising	Dried figs or fresh fruit or dry fruit *1 tsp of gulkand	Nuts are a good source of magnesium so are fresh fruits like banana. *If acidity is bad, delay the fruit by 20-30 mins, start with gulkand and give the body time to settle down.
Meal 2 – Breakfast / within 90 mins	Ragi satva or daliya *Kadak pav and butter or *Poha or jowar flakes and milk	Complete meal, good start to the day. *Options when very acidic or nauseous.

Timing	Meals	Notes
Meal 3 – Mid-morning	Kokum sherbet / nariyal pani and malai	Reduces acidity, bloating and detoxes.
Meal 4 – Lunch / Between 11 a.m. and 1 p.m. + Vit D 1000IU	Ragi roti / jowar roti + sabzi + chaas with *Hingashtak or **Dahi-rice-sabzi	Add 1 tsp of ghee to the roti / bhakri. Either keep ghee in office or add at home. Avoids afternoon slump and post-lunch craving. *Hingashtak is hing mixed with herbs and salts, especially useful for the gut bacteria. **If very acidic.
Meal 5 - Mid-meal/ 3 pm	Handful of peanuts and chana or fresh fruit or homemade laddoo	Can have chai / coffee here with this meal. Add ginger or lemon grass if feeling low or acidic. If drinking chai in office, ensure that chai powder is not getting reused for your cuppa.
Meal 6 – 5 to 6 p.m. + Vit B with folic acid	Egg and toast or chutney toast or banana or poha or fresh fruit milkshake	Very important meal, to keep the cortisol levels down and prevent protein losses. An on-the-go meal. Once a week, homemade deep-fried snack here.

Timing	Meals	Notes
Meal 7 – dinner / 7 to 8.30 p.m. + Vit C 500mg	Khichdi + boiled beet / ragi dosa with paneer bhurji / lentils and rice + homemade pickle *Rice pej with ghee	Easy to digest and nutritious meal. Plan for Meal 6 and 7 ideally a week in advance. Husbands, cook dinner at least two times a week, preferably pre-decided days as per wife's convenience. *Acidic or very sick.
Meal 8 – If needed + Bedtime calcium citrate 1000mg	Cup of milk with haldi	Serves as a nightcap and the haldi works as an anti-inflammatory agent, improves your chances of reduced morning sickness the next day.

Important notes for T1

- Use your regional alternatives whenever possible.

- Get yourself the most local variety of the fruit. E.g. the red banana if you can, or at least the small yellow one. The local jamun, bor, seetaphal, mango, jackfruit, guava, depending on what is in season.

- Avoid the exotic vegetables and fruits — avocado, kale, kiwi, blueberries, etc.

- Don't eat raw veggies other than raw tomato, onion

and cucumber, and even then only as a small part of the meal. Eat with lunch and not with dinner unless it's prepared as koshimbir or raita.

- Eat sabzi of raw banana, suran, arbi, sweet potato — veggies of this category — at least twice a week to support the T1 hormones and keep acidity down.

- If you feel like chaat or something fried, Meal 6 is a good place, and as far as possible make it at home.

- Preferable laddoos — rava nariyal or besan or ragi laddoo

- Kadak pav or poee is the bread that is bought from a local bakery, invariably richer in Vit B than the mass-made variety.

- Supplements are kept for the latter half of the day as nausea (if existing) will usually settle post lunch.

- Drink enough water to stay hydrated and always check that urine is crystal clear.

- Pickle should be homemade or made in the home of a trusted source and with unrefined salt, not the white one.

- Ghee can be homemade or bought from a small goshala (which has desi cows) and not mass manufactured to ensure authenticity of source and to get the right essential fatty acids from it.

HERITAGE RECIPES FOR T1

The heritage recipes have been contributed by people from across India (and also Indians across the globe), and follow the basics of the core principles of eating right during and post pregnancy. They are easy, quick, nutritious and most importantly, time-tested. They are also a representation of hundreds of similar homemade recipes and ingredients across regions, communities and households. Relish them.

Recipe 1: Ghee rice — Neychoru (Kerala)

Contributed by Rakhi Vinay, Kerala / Canada

Rujuta says: This is a cooling meal and has ingredients that act as a natural antacid.

Stepwise instructions:

- Add homemade ghee to the kadai.
- Once the ghee starts to melt, add shallots (small onions) cut into halves. Sauté until you get a golden brown tinge and a great smell. This takes up to 10 minutes.
- Slowly add boiled rice into this mixture and mix well.

PREGNANCY NOTES

- Add curry leaves.
- Put the heat off. Serve it hot.

Recipe 2: *Murakakerai saag (Drumstick leaves)*

Contributed by Richa Rungta, Chennai

Rujuta says: A mineral-rich sabzi, the drumstick, or moringa, will help prevent calcium losses and keep Hb levels high.

Stepwise instructions:
- Take 1 bowl of drumstick leaves and one chopped onion.
- Heat 1 small tsp of homemade ghee in a kadai.
- Add jeera and 1 Kashmiri mirch for the fragrance.
- Add chopped onion and sauté it for 5 minutes.
- Add salt as per taste.
- Add the drumstick leaves and sauté for 5 minutes.
- Turn off the gas. Eat it with rice or wheat roti.

This vegetable relieves you from any pain in the body during pregnancy, and also your baby gets good hair and you are hydrated throughout the day.

| 79 |

Recipe 3: Panchamrit

Contributed by Muktai Khandekar Badarayani, New York

Rujuta says: This is one of your hyper local, secret recipes that helps keep your hormones in a state of balance.

Stepwise instructions:

- Take one silver bowl, clean it thoroughly.
- Add 1 tsp honey, 1 tsp curd, 1 tsp sugar, 2 tsp cow ghee, 7-8 tsp milk (boiled and then cooled down to room temperature), and one strip of kesar (saffron).
- Mix and keep in the silver bowl overnight.
- After you freshen up, eat this first thing in the morning for its good assimilation.

Tip:

1. Do not use hot milk. Curd being one of the ingredients, the whole thing might turn into curd after you keep it overnight.
2. You can also use this preparation as a base for massaging your dry skin (especially on dry nipples

which happens often during pregnancy).

Recipe 4: Beet raita

Contributed by Ankita Diwekar Kabra, Surat

Rujuta says: A nutrient-rich recipe that's easy to cook and an alternative to cooking sabzis. Can be easily made by husband without goofing up.

Stepwise instructions:

1. Take 2 cups of boiled, peeled and mashed beetroot.

2. Add a cup of fresh curd to it and mix together.

3. Add salt, a pinch of sugar, chopped coriander and 2 chopped green chillies to the beetroot and curd mixture.

4. Heat 1 tsp of ghee in a small tempering pan. Add asafoetida and jeera to the ghee till it splutters.

5. Pour the tempering mixture over the raita and mix well.

Recipe 5: Suranache kaap (Yam)

Contributed by Rujuta Diwekar

Have added this so that husbands can contribute in

the kitchen. The wife is not going to feel like a full-fledged meal, so she can eat this instead of nothing or just the 'kaap' instead of sabzi with either dahi-rice or just rice.

Stepwise instructions:

Suranache kaap (yam is called suran in Marathi) is a great starter by itself. It is traditionally served as an accompaniment with a hot meal of dal-chawal.

1. Roughly cut the outer skin of the yam with a sharp knife.
2. Chop the yam in big chunks / blocks.
3. Pressure cook the yam blocks and then allow to cool completely.
4. Slice the yam into ¼ inch-thick long pieces. .
5. Shallow fry in oil on a cast-iron tava till the yam slices turn crispy on both sides.
6. Season with salt and red chilli powder.
7. Serve hot.

You can make 'kaap' with raw bananas and potatoes too. For these three, skip the pressure cooking step. You need to marinate the sliced vegetable with salt, turmeric and red chilli powder half an hour beforehand. Coat the sliced vegetables with rava (semolina) or rice flour before shallow frying.

Special Note on Iron Supplementation

One of the standard operating procedures is to put all pregnant women on an iron tab, but the question is, is that really necessary? Well, if you look at scientific data, then the answer is no. Pregnancy is a time when a woman is at her most vulnerable phase and this exposes her to many half-baked truths. It's not unusual for doctors to stop all the vitamin supplements that you were on and to start you exclusively on iron, folic acid and calcium. And it's even less unusual for us to actually question that, so here's some much needed education on iron absorption and assimilation.

Pregnant and lactating women need about 20-30 mg of iron per day to bear the physiological stresses. Anaemia or low Hb levels will make it harder for the body to carry oxygen and nutrients and leave you feeling tired and exhausted. It will also put you at a risk of developing infections and could cause low birth weight for the baby. However, all this is likely to happen if the anaemia lasts for a very long time and the Hb levels are really low, like 9 and under.

The levels to aim for are 11 and above pre-pregnancy, post-delivery and for the first trimester. As you get into the second trimester, 10.5 gm per decilitre is considered a normal level. This is because the blood volume is enlarged and Hb is measured as a concentration.

When the volume is high, concentration is low. If you are at these levels and popping a pill, know that it is bringing no benefit to the body. A well-documented fact about iron supplementation is that it works when the levels are fairly low (7–9 and at even lower levels you may need transfusion). The iron pills come with their side effects of constipation, diarrhoea, nausea and vomiting, so why add to your already existing morning sickness? This note and, in fact, the book is to ensure that you are making informed decisions based on facts, not fads and much worse, fears.

Absorption and assimilation of iron is helped by certain co-factors and your lifestyle. Here are things that you can do:

- Vitamin C is a co-factor in absorption of iron, so fresh fruits like peru and cashew fruit as well as amla murabbas, nimbu sherbet, etc., aid assimilation. Vit C increases iron availability up to three times.

- Vit B12 is a co-factor too, so dahi, chaas, even homemade dhokla, kadhis are good sources, not to forget the achaars that help keep the gut bacteria and promote assimilation of nutrients from food.

- Precursors of Vit A, like carotenes, help assimilation of iron too and, therefore, the traditional suggestion of sweet potato, pumpkin, and local fruits like seetaphal and ramphal.

- Seeds rich in essential fats and minerals — essentially the stuff that we use in tadka like rai, jeera and even til seeds, seeds from doodhi, pumpkin help.

- Cooking in iron kadais and on an iron tava helps you assimilate iron better and enriches the iron content of every meal.

- Nuts and dry fruits are an important source not just of iron but of other essential nutrients and co-factors. Start with a handful every day or have them as a mid-day snack. Peanuts and jaggery and coconut is a wonderful meal too.

- Above all, exercise and sleep are important as they promote healthy mucus membrane for the intestines, keep the diversity and strength of the friendly bacteria and much more importantly, make every cell of the body more sensitive to nutrients.

- And don't forget to eat in silver thalis and katoris. Bring them out of your locker, as other than helping with iron assimilation, they also help prevent infections and allergies.

The stuff that comes in the way of iron absorption (and if you have these, popping a pill doesn't help either):

- A diet that is poor in all of the above nutrients.

- A very common approach of vegetarians is to eat an egg as a form of protein during pregnancy, but the thing is that eggs actually contain a compound called phosvitin that inhibits iron absorption. This is called the egg factor. Basically, don't change your diet pattern and change from vegetarian to non-vegetarian or vice versa, because in the hope of getting one nutrient, you could be losing out on another, or worse, on many others.

- Smoking, or second-hand smoking, is a big hindrance so avoid that at all costs.

- Taking photon inhibitors, antacids (commonly used to treat morning sickness), interfere with iron absorption.

- Lack of exercise, a sedentary lifestyle and poor sleep are the big factors that prevent assimilation of iron.

- Consumption of packaged and processed foods including fibre-rich cereals, biscuits, breads, etc.

- Coffee, chocolates and the green teas with polyphenols that you are dousing yourself in as healthy are iron absorption inhibitors too.

- Spinach, btw, is not such a great source. Iron from spinach and the other raw juices that you drink (for their nutrient-rich properties) comes in a bound form and it is difficult for the body to absorb iron from these sources. So much for your green– and red-coloured juices. Cooking sabzis helps release the bound vitamins though.

Essentially, stick to traditional diets, regulate your lifestyle and ensure that you are not a victim of nutrition transition. One where you give up on your grandmom's diet and follow the tabloid and fashion mag diet (Western diet is what it is called in scientific literature), and land up with the 'big mother, small baby' syndrome; where babies are 3 kgs and lower and mothers have gained up to 25 kgs in pregnancy.

THE SECOND TRIMESTER (T2)

'I hated the fact that Navin had his hands on my tummy. "Oh, I can't feel anything," said the idiot. The baby doesn't like you, I said. "Must be a boy then," he replied. I hated Navin and his type, the middle-aged men who thought they were teens, wrapping their hands around pregnant women as if they were up for grabs. The problem was I liked Navin's wife as much as I disliked him. She was by the bar sipping wine. "Iram, the fact is I haven't felt any movement." "Then really must be a boy, lazy from the womb," she said, throwing her head back, roaring with laughter. After laughing she usually gets serious and gives out gyaan, so I waited for her to finish. "Listen, it's barely what? Eighteen weeks? That's nothing. In the first one, it takes time, twenty-two weeks or maybe even twenty-five. Check with Madhu." My gyny and her friend, Madhu had told me the same thing last week, but now that Iram had said it, I believed it. There is something special about women who live with idiotic men: they give you the truth to your face and you can always trust them.'

Questions for T2 then:
FAQs for T2

1. Is it safe for me to work out now?

Not just ultra safe but ultra recommended that you start working out now, if you haven't already, or were having a particularly bad time during T1. The key is to start with small steps, keep the workout to a small duration of twenty-thirty minutes, and at all times stay in the comfortable but not lazy zone. Working out under the supervision of an experienced and well-informed trainer is especially useful during this time and worth the investment. Babies of mommies who exercise are born leaner and with a better immune system.

Work out up to three to five days a week depending on your comfort level, and keep the activity levels high through the day. Stand for three minutes for every thirty minutes of sitting, walk around the office / home as often as you can, or go for a light walk of twenty minutes every day.

Not exercising and sitting around, or worse, lying around all day will reduce your insulin sensitivity, reduce the anabolic stimuli (protein synthesis and assimilation) and make you vulnerable to developing hormonal imbalances. The risk of gestational diabetes or post-delivery thyroid is especially high if you are unfit / inactive. So every little step counts.

Moreover, exercise also means better blood circulation, better digestion, and it has a natural hypotensive (blood pressure reducing) effect too. So move, don't sit, you are pregnant, not sick.

2. I have been put on bed rest by my doc, what now?

Speak to your doc and figure out if the bed rest is really critical or is it in response to your or your family's hyper behaviour. Also, engage with a doctor who is willing to talk to you, answer your questions and is appreciative of the fact that it may be routine for her / him, but for you this is make or break. Have Kangana's attitude and learn from what she said on Karan Johar's show — her director shouldn't be a dictator but someone who sees it as a collaboration. Know that your smooth delivery reflects well on your doc's résumé too. If your doc is a dictator, drop him and find another one; the last thing you need right now is stress.

The lecture apart, know that bed rest will lead to a drop in insulin sensitivity and make you further prone to complications. Ask your doc whether you can stand often, walk around a bit — the answer to this is yes most of the time. And if it's a complete no, ask if it's for a few days or does your doc envision this to be your state for the next few months all the way to your delivery. And if you really can't do anything but be in bed all day, then move your muscles, contract and relax them while lying down so that at least some stimuli is being provided. And though you cannot completely undo the damage that the body will go through, at least you are limiting it, and can be back to rebuilding the tone and fitness in the body in a couple of months post delivery.

Hint: if your doc is saying that you can walk to the loo, then it means that light movement for the body where you are not unduly exerting yourself is not going to hurt. Also remember, movement / activity / exercise is critical for better blood flow to the foetus, keeping your BP down and preventing piles and constipation.

3. Is there a yoga routine you recommend?

If you already have a yoga teacher, continue with what she / he teaches you. The pregnancy guide, *Iyengar Yoga for Motherhood*, is an excellent resource. Mumbai, I feel, is especially lucky, because we have pregnancy classes at Iyengar yoga centres, where you find women doing various asanas and the routine changes according to the stage of pregnancy you are in. Of course, it's important to exercise caution at all times, and therefore, investing time in travelling to a class where the teacher is well trained and experienced, or investing money in a book that teaches you exactly how to do it, is well worth the buck. With *Iyengar Yoga for Motherhood*, you have your bases covered: it has sequences for acidity, diabetes, mental stability and a trimester by trimester sequence with detailed instructions and photographs.

4. Can I travel right now?

Universally, this is supposed to be a good time to

travel, and people even have babymoons during these months. Stay well hydrated on the journey as long air travel can be dehydrating, and if you are driving, take frequent breaks as sitting for too long can be a bummer for the back. Choose places that serve good food, as eating right is critical. Also, do not try new cuisines, or seafood, or raw salads while outside. Preferably, go to a place you have already been to as it's familiar territory and you know what to expect; also, it will be easier to have your special requirements accommodated. Avoid places that have bars on the property as the smoke or loud noise could be disturbing, and choose cities where outdoor smoking is not a thing so that you don't land up with some throat infection or get sick just because of the holiday.

5. My mother-in-law is insisting I have halwa and laddoos. Should I?

Absolutely, please do. Have them mid-morning or mid-afternoon and know that if the battle is between the dietician and your grandmother, dadi / nani wins, hands down, every time. And probably we will add what she told you in the next edition of this book.

6. The constipation is killing me. What to do?

Do this:

- Warm glass of water before every meal.
- Half tsp of gulkand after every meal.
- Vit B6 with dinner.

And you should be sorted.

7. What to do for backache?

The food and exercise should take care of it, but here are few things you can try:

- Learn to stand correctly so that the weight is well balanced on your two feet.
- Increase the strength of your adductors, inner thighs. When at home, you can press a block between your thighs. Pay special attention to them during your yoga practice.
- Work at improving the flexibility in your hamstrings.
- Use a footstool for your legs in office.
- Drink enough water, cut down on tea / coffee / colas.

- Stand often and don't sit in one place for too long.

- Try the sequence for the back from the *Iyengar Yoga for Motherhood* book.

- Take a calcium supplement.

The Top Three Foods for T2

Though this is officially the easiest time of the pregnancy, this is also the period that is going to decide how smooth your delivery is and how quickly you get back in shape post it.

> It's officially the time to increase the essential fat in the diet, for many reasons; the main one would be to improve insulin sensitivity and to strengthen the joints and prevent backaches.

And without the support of essential fatty acids and the fat-soluble vitamins that come with it, Vit A, D, E, K, changes to the skin and hair can occur too. So T2 is actually nature's way to give you the time to have everything in your control before any damage — stretch marks, loss of hair, pigmentation, etc. — can take place.

And to do this job are nature's very own beauty pills — the ones that keep blood sugars under control, help improve bone and joint health and provide the amino acids that keep the skin supple and fresh. Here we go:

T2F1: *Nutmeg or Jaiphal*

This spice is used in tiny amounts to flavour kheer, halwas and laddoos. Rich in antioxidant properties and minerals, jaiphal is used to improve digestion, prevent hair loss and fine lines or wrinkling of the skin, and to reduce blood pressure. The key though, as with any spice, is to use it intelligently, that is in amounts that are tiny enough to just hint at the presence of the spice. Because it's exactly in these amounts that it is medicinal. It even helps in the production of red blood cells and keeps fatigue away.

How to use it:

- Flavouring agent in laddoos, kheer, halwa.
- Mixed with besan and milk, applied to the skin to help achieve a smooth skin and prevent itching (especially for itchy nipples or thighs).
- Add a pinch to milk and have it at bedtime for better sleep.

T2F2: Ghee

Ah! You were waiting for this one. From the short chain fatty acids that help the intestines function better and support the growth of the good bacteria to helping accelerate fat-burning and making food delicious, ghee is truly the most divine fat on earth. Its benefits are many; one of the most important ones during pregnancy is that the addition of ghee to food slows down the rate at which blood sugars climb and this quality really helps support both the thyroid and the insulin hormone. The key here is to make it from full fat milk from indigenous (desi) cows, and if not desi cows, then buffalos, but never Jersey or Holstein cows. Make it at home, and if not home, buy from a trustworthy, small gaushala.

How to use it:

- Add a tsp or two to your rotis and rice. If there is a history of diabetes in the family, add a little extra, as the addition of essential fat helps support the insulin function.

- You can use it for tadka or cooking of dals, sabzis and biryanis. And of course in laddoos, halwa or barfis.

- Rub the soles of your feet with ghee in the night to prevent constipation and induce better sleep.

T2F3: *Foxtail millet / Kangani / Tenai/ Rala / Koralu*

Since millets grow across India, you will have local names based on the region you come from. The foxtail millet looks like couscous or tiny grains of rice or rava and is cooked exactly the way you would make rice. From upma to pulao to kheer, it blends quite well in all regional recipes. It tastes especially nice when made with peanuts or cooked like plain rice and eaten with lentils. It's known to reduce blood sugars and c-reactive protein (something that rises when inflammation or BP rises), and like all millets helps improve the HDL levels.

How to use it:

- Cook like rice and eat it with lentils or dals.

- Can be sprouted and made into malt / porridge which makes vitamin B more available. Or make it like a kheer with dry fruits.

- Make it like a dalia or an upma with veggies and peas.

The T2 Meal Plan

Meal Timings	Meals	Notes
Meal 1 – Within 15 mins of waking up	Fresh fruit /dry fruit / overnight soaked black raisins	Make a serious effort to get more active. Stand, walk around the house for 10-15 mins.
Meal 2 – Breakfast / within 60 mins + Vit B with folic acid or pregnancy vitamin	Any homemade nashta / foxtail upma with veggies	You can carry this to office as lunch too.
Meal 3 – Mid-morning	Nariyal pani with malai / laddoo with til / peanuts / rajgeera chiki	Mixture of jaggery with nuts that are rich in essential fatty acids to keep blood sugars regulated, skin supple, joints strong.
Meal 4 – Lunch + Flaxseed or ALA supplement	Foxtail millet cooked like rice mixed with dal / upma made with peanuts *Ragi or wheat roti with sabzi + beetroot or doodhi raita	Wholesome meals that will keep you energetic through the day. *Add two tsp of ghee to this meal, you now need higher amounts of essential fats.

Meal Timings	Meals	Notes
Meal 5 – Mid-afternoon	Chaas with hingashtak and kalanamak or laddoo or chiki like Meal 3	Choose the meal as per appetite.
Meal 6 – Between 5 and 6 p.m. + Vit C 500mg, antioxidant with selenium, zinc, chromium	Ragi dosa with til or coconut chutney / ragi satva with pinch of jaiphal / sandwich with coconut and til chutney / roti with chutney or jaggery and ghee / fresh fruit: banana or mango (if it's in season) / * whey protein shake	Wholesome meal to keep the hormones in a state of balance and reduce the chances of bloating and constipation. Plan for a workout before this meal if possible. Or an hour after this meal, just pre-dinner. *Have the whey protein only if you have been having it in pre-pregnancy state.
Meal 7 – Dinner	Dal rice + achaar / khichdi and kadhi + boiled beets / veg pulao + veggies	Keep the dinner light and easy to digest. Add 2 tsp of ghee to dinner.
Meal 8 – If needed + bedtime calcium citrate 1000 mg	Milk + pinch of jaiphal + 3-4 soaked kaju + sugar to taste	If hungry and if sleep is disturbed or you are mentally too tired or if there are digestion issues.

Important Notes for T2

- *Foxtail is easy to find online or in organic stores around your area. If you have never had it, once or twice a week is a good start and you can have regular roti / rice on other days.*

- *Buy whole gehu and then have it made into a flour in a local chakki. Avoid buying readymade attas.*

- *When choosing bread, avoid multigrain breads as there is a method to mixing grains often ignored in commercial breads. E.g. bajra is best consumed exclusively in winter and its consumption during summer may leave you heavy and dehydrated.*

- *If you are put on a protein drink, do read the label and ensure that you are not consuming tons of sugar to get a few grams of protein. Most health or 'for mother' drinks have a profile of 2:1 of carb to protein. That's a poor ratio and you are better off avoiding those.*

- *If you need more protein in your diet but have never taken whey protein before, take half a scoop of whey in water and drink it with lunch / dinner to support protein intake. And if you feel uncomfortable, discontinue.*

- *Always remember that the way to get more protein is to provide the anabolic stimuli: stay active, exercise, sleep on time and eat often.*

- If you are constipated or suffering from digestion issues, have a glass of warm water before breakfast, lunch and dinner.

- If the constipation problem is persistent, have milk with gulkand either as Meal 6 or Meal 8. Don't worry about sugar in the gulkand, you will be well within the six to nine tsp of sugar / day limit if you go by the plan.

- Keep the rice white or single-polished and buy the local variety.

- Moong dal khichdi is a good alternative to any of the big meals, and is easy to prepare. Allow people at home to help out in the kitchen.

- If you are a husband who can totally not cook, ensure that before and after cooking there is absolutely nothing that your wife needs to look into. Clean up before and after, and if you have help at home, ensure that they direct questions to you and not your wife. If you live with your mum, then make sure that the job your wife was doing earlier is not being transferred to Mummyji and that you are able to put your mum at ease and do those tasks yourself. Ya, we are treating you like an adult.

- If you are a mom whose heart breaks at the sight of your son in the kitchen, breathe. You did a better job at raising him than your MIL did with her son, your husband. Besides boys who are active in the kitchen earn more gratitude and sexual favours from their wives. Relax, he knows what he is doing.

· Again, eat a variety of fruits — keep them local.

· In addition to the sabzis of T1, eat leafy veggies if they are in season (winter) and ensure that you are eating the indigenous veggies that grow on creepers twice a week — pumpkin, doodhi, gourds of all kinds.

· The creeper veggies are indigenous and require no fertilizers or pesticides for their growth. Besides, they are great source of the micro-minerals that your body needs to keep blood sugars, BP and moods steady.

· Stay well hydrated, make sure that your urine is clear.

VEG OR NON-VEG DURING / POST PREGNANCY

The big trend in nutrition science for 2017 (and a much-needed one) is sustainability. One where vegetarians don't eat eggs or fish or other meat products to get more protein. And one where non-vegetarian communities eat the way their grandmother taught them to — meat / fish a few times a week, not every day, not at every meal and only as a part of the whole meal; with rice or bhakri / roti, along with the sabzi, etc. This is a sustainable way of eating, good for preventing diseases and also climate change. Your grandmom knew, her grandmom knew too, but nutrition societies are just discovering it, and the likes of Jamie Oliver are posting #meatlessmonday recipes every week and USA and Swiss Olympic associations are regulating meat intake of super athletes. Regarding pregnancy, the only time you should avoid meat is in the first twelve days post delivery.

And while talking about meat, what about milk and milk products? Again, they are an integral part of both our local economy and of creating a sustainable environment too. Patronize the desi cow, and if you are rich enough, raise some cows; they are our original pets (not dogs), in fact, our wealth. Desi cow milk, with its unique protein and fatty acid profile, helps prevent diabetes, bone losses and skin pigmentation. The reports you read of milk doing terrible stuff to the body is not coming from the indigenous variety of Indian or African cows. And the mass milking where four udders are milked is not how Indian farmers milk the cow. If you were taught the basics of farming in school, or taken to a village early in life, then you would know that a cow is milked only from two udders and two are for the calf. And that if the calf drinks too much milk (and there is such a thing) then it gets looseys. So no, cruelty (towards cows and calves) is not a desi concept.

Heritage Recipes for T2

Recipe 1: Banana flower curry (Koldil bhaji)

Contributed by Ruhi Sahu, Assam

Rujuta says: You almost go into a meditative state while cleaning up the banana flower.

Stepwise instructions:

Remove the outer elongated red leaf of the banana flower and pluck the small white flowers that are inside. Keep removing the leaves and pluck all the flowers till done.

- In a pan, put oil.
- Once oil is hot, add bay leaf, chopped onions, tomatoes and ginger-garlic paste.
- Once the onion starts to sweat, add small cubes of potatoes.
- Add cumin powder, turmeric powder, coriander powder and salt.
- Add banana flowers to the pan. Mix it well and add water. Cover the pan with a lid and let it cook for 20 minutes.
- After 15 minutes, add curry patta and poppy seeds and let it cook for 5 to 10 minutes more.
- Remove from the pan and garnish with coriander and green chilli.

Recipe 2: Raw chalimidi

Contributed by Madduri Sai, Hyderabad

Rujuta says: Rice, the eternal grain of growth, is used here to both break the news to others and to help the young mommy stay calm.

Stepwise instructions:

- Soak rice overnight and grind it to make rice flour.
- Add grated coconut, jaggery syrup / sugar and ghee to the rice flour.
- Make it into a thick dough and keep it aside for 60 minutes and then make small balls and eat.

The mother prepares and makes the pregnant daughter eat this in the third month and then the news is shared with everyone (twelfth week). Also, after delivery, when the girl leaves for the in-laws' place, chalimidi is put in a cloth and tied to the stomach.

Recipe 3: Coconut mishri

Contributed by Monika Agrawal, Rajasthan

Rujuta says: The lauric acid in coconut is an anti-bacterial, anti-fungal and anti-viral agent. It's also one of the main ingredients of breast milk.

Stepwise instructions:

- 1 bowl crushed sukha coconut.
- 1 bowl mishri, crushed or coarsely chopped.

- Mix the above together and take it whenever you feel like. Best in the early morning, before breakfast.

It gives relief from bloating and good growth to the foetus. As a custom, the mother gives this to the pregnant daughter so that her grandchild has smooth skin and hair.

Recipe 4: Badami lehya

Contributed by Aishwarya A. Narayan, Bangalore

Rujuta says: This is the original essential fatty acid supplement, the one that belongs to our collective wisdom about food.

Stepwise instructions:

- Blend the red stone sugar (kallu shakare) to a fine powder.
- Mix it with a little water so that it dissolves and start heating it in a thick vessel.
- Grind the badam to a fine powder and mix it to the sugar syrup.
- Keep stirring and add ghee simultaneously.
- Add kesar and stir till the consistency is like a

thick ball leaving the sides of the vessel. This takes approximately 20 to 25 minutes.

- After this, add elaichi powder and switch off the flame.
- After it completely cools, store in an airtight box.

Can be consumed every day first thing in the morning. It works wonders.

Recipe 5: Drumstick aamti

Contributed by Renuka Omkar Saraf, Sangamner

Rujuta says: A local delicacy that will help keep the acidity and bloating down. It's a nutrient super power of sorts.

Stepwise instructions:

1. Boil drumsticks in water with salt.
2. Roast dry coconut, khus khus and a little jeera and grind to a fine paste. Add some water.
3. Heat oil in pan / kadhai, add hing, halad and the ground paste.
4. Stir and add boiled drumsticks into it. Add salt to taste.

You can eat it with bhakri or roti and do not forget to take 2 tsp of sajuk tup with it.

Recipe 6: Ambehaldi che lonche (Turmeric and ginger relish)

Contributed by Rujuta Diwekar

Again, easy-to-cook and best made by husbands. This one ensures that your skin stays smooth and hydrated through the pregnancy and helps prevent infections too.

Stepwise instructions:

There are two varieties of fresh turmeric available. One is called 'ambe halad' or 'mango ginger'. It looks very similar to fresh ginger or adrak, but has the rich, yellow colour of a ripe mango. The other variant is called 'oli halad', or white turmeric. This looks very similar to fresh ginger. This relish recipe calls for ginger, chillies and both variants of fresh turmeric. A perfect, tangy accompaniment to your meal!

1. Take equal quantities of mango ginger, white turmeric and fresh ginger. Wash, peel and cut in short, thin strips.

2. Take a few green chillies, split midway, remove the seeds and cut in short, thin strips.

3. To this mixture, add lemon juice, pickle masala and salt.

4. Separately, heat oil and add mustard seeds, asafoetida and dry turmeric powder.

5. Allow the tadka mixture to cool down completely and then pour it over the ginger, turmeric and chilli mixture.

You can make this relish and store it for up to two months in the refrigerator or make it fresh every few days. It can be had throughout your pregnancy.

THE THIRD TRIMESTER (T3)

'If there's one thing I couldn't imagine life without, it was work, and I had it all planned around my work life. Who to marry, where to live, and when to get pregnant. IIM-A should be giving me a medal or calling me to speak in a class that teaches women to keep and rock at their careers post-marriage. I had it all under my control: there were boundaries that my mother-in-law and mother had learnt not to cross; my bosses had learnt not to push me aside for important foreign travel just because I was an expectant mother. But the one thing I couldn't control was the bloody traffic. Powai to JVLR was taking longer than expected and I had timed my pee in such a way that I could just about make it home, park, take the elevator and open two doors — house and then bathroom — to finally do it. But today, my carefully planned arithmetic was coming apart and I was losing control of my bladder. I hadn't peed in my stretch pants yet, but I could feel the heaviness and I jumped the signal on amber near Renaissance Hotel. I shouldn't have — my equation had already accounted for a cop there — but like I told you, I was losing control today.

'The cop waved me down but nothing, not even the law (my law-abiding parents and society in Bhilai would be ashamed of me), was going to stop me today. I zoomed past the cop and before I knew it he was on his bike chasing me. It was straight out of some action movie, I drove at speeds I had no idea my car could do and he made some solid swerves to catch up with me. Just when I thought I had made it, he caught up with me, parked his bike in front of my car and was tapping on my window.

'I gave up and rolled my window down. "Pagal hai kya?" he asked. Pregnant hai, I answered, zor ka sussu aa raha hai. His face fell and I heard him say, "Sorry madam, you took risk because of me. Sorry madam, apna country cashless ho gaya par abhi tak ladies log ke liye toilet nahi hai." Or at least I think he said something like that, because by then I had lost all my hard-gained control — over emotions, life, and even my bladder. I was sobbing uncontrollably, making sounds I had never heard before, unbelievable na? The steering wheel could no longer take the weight of my face and it blew the horn, literally. "Kisi ko phone karu madam? Address kya hai?" Sir, I said, wiping my tears and gaining some control over my voice, it's okay I am close by, I will go. He walked back to his bike, made way for my car, and followed from a distance till I turned into my building.'

Phew, let's move on to the questions:
FAQs for T3

1. Listen, I just can't sleep. What should I do?

It's not unusual to get all angsty and impatient in the last few weeks, but just because you want it out, it is not going to come out (you knew that, sorry for stating the obvious). The thing is, it's a tender state for the hormones to be in. That extra cup of coffee post 4 p.m., the teeny chocolate you bit into post lunch, the irritation you felt at your MIL's WhatsApp dp is all going to cost you your sleep. And without sleep, you will feel bloated, annoyed and generally low, so do yourself a favour — keep calm and sleep it off. Here are a few things that help:

- Practise unhearing every bit of random advice that's coming your way.

- Work at eating in silence and with your hands. It helps you better connect with your satiety signals.

- Regulate gadget use. Give yourself a fixed thirty minutes every day on your phone to check social media status or to play stupid games, no more. And surely not after dinner.

- Kokum butter to the soles of your feet, nasal ghee drops and ghee mixed with ajwain applied on the stomach will work wonders for restorative sleep.

- A glass of milk with soaked cashews, haldi and jaiphal is a great nightcap as well as a hormone regulator and immunity booster. Helps cut down bloating too.

- Nap for twenty minutes in the afternoon to help the body unwind, but not any longer.

- Keep your body and bedroom cool. Turn the AC on before you hit the bed — that way you are not lying there waiting for the cooling to kick in.

- Exercise. The blood circulation and hormonal balance it brings about is a sleep regulator too.

2. How will I know if it's real and not false labour?

It's easy to interpret every contraction as labour pain,

especially if it's your first time. A good doctor will help you tell the difference, so have a relaxed conversation with her / him to help understand if it's really the time. Ideally, the later you reach the hospital, the better, because the gyny is not going to see you till you are totally dilated and the nurses and sisters are not going to take grief from you while you are in the process either. So my advice is, instead of talking to your doctor about other things, ask her / him to tell you honestly when you should get to the hospital.

3. I might have gestational diabetes. Should I start the diabetes pill?

- Before you decide that you have gestational diabetes (GDM) look for other clinical parameters — what are the triglycerides looking like? What about Vit B12 and Vit D status? Are there signs of low energy or inflammation? Is there a history of complications during pregnancy? If everything is within range, it could just be one random reading.

- If all other parameters are within range, then ask for another test of GCT (glucose challenge test, a shorter version of OGTT), and if you have eaten right and gotten a workout, it's most likely to come within range.

- A hypoglycaemic (blood sugar lowering) drug is going to both disturb the gut bacteria and assimilation of Vit B12 and D. So ensure that you have not left any stone unturned before popping the pill.

- Sleeping well and de-stressing is crucial for the sugars to stabilize, so don't fight the husband or the boss; relax. You being edgy will hurt you more than these people.

- Hold a glass of milk at bedtime in your hands and ditch the gadget. While reading off your smart phone will do silly things to your blood sugars, a glass of milk with its amino acid and essential fatty acid profile will help them stay steady.

- Lastly, know that fear and anxiety is also a hindrance to the body's ability to stabilize blood sugars. So don't fear the worst; know that GDM is totally preventable and responds beautifully to lifestyle modifications.

4. My doc says I am prone to blood sugar issues, what can I do?

Do this:

- Add ghee to your chapati or dal-chawal so that the sugars climb slowly.

- Improve the nutrient content of your meal — eat wholesome and include legumes and millets in your daily diet.

- Break up your meals into smaller portions and chew well.

- Add essential fats to your diet: til chutney, sunflower seed chutney, peanut chutney, a little achaar — one of these with lunch and dinner.

- Coconut laddoos, til or peanut chiki or paneer or nuts as mid-meals to further help steady the sugars.

- Move more, workout even if it's a light one as exercise improves insulin sensitivity and glucose uptake by the cells. The effect will last up to seventy-two hours.

- Work at eating the forgotten local foods as

they are richer in micro-nutrients like folic acid, Vit B12 and minerals. These help improve iron status and nutrient assimilation, which in turn helps lower the blood sugars.

5. Should I start jhadu-katka of my house or at least my room for ease of delivery?

We have to see the jhadu-katka thing in better perspective. At one time, this was a regular activity for women and the message here really is to keep up with your regular activity. Today, for us, 'regular' is going to work, doing our daily chores, blow-drying our hair ;) — essentially, keeping up with one's routine and getting on with one's life instead of holding your breath for the big day is the key here. So, if jhadu-katka is not in your routine, don't do it.

6. How soon before I get back in shape?

For starters, being in shape has nothing to do with size but how well you feel from within. You will be back to your non-pregnant shape once you deliver and you will fit into all your pre-pregnancy clothes within four to six months of having the baby. Your baby itself will be about 3-4 kgs; 4 kgs is just the extra fluids and blood volume, about 2 kgs is the placenta and uterus, 1 kg of extra breast tissue and between 1-4 kgs is the extra fat and nutrients that your body carries. Other than the fat, expect most of the weight to come off at the delivery table. And the fat can go slowly, but at this point it is of paramount importance for the health of both you and your baby. It boosts the immune system, provides for extra cushioning and helps in thermo-regulation and lactation post-delivery. The idea is to not rush the process and shed the weight; the body is meant to change, celebrate it like Kareena did.

7. Should I shave my pubic hair?

A lot of hospitals do that for you, or you can have it done in the comfort of your home before you go to deliver.

8. I am scared, will everything be okay for my baby?

Totally, nature is on your baby's side. Nothing untoward is likely to happen, so breathe and be happy.

Top Three Foods for T3

T3 can be a tiring phase and a test of patience, literally. On the one hand you want to let it all go, on the other you are constantly aware that once you do let go, nothing will ever be the same again. The baby will change your life forever, and other than her health, security and well-being, nothing else will matter. The next six months can be quite overwhelming — the delivery, the ability to feed, the staying up in the nights, the warding off of random advice and the scepticism about whether the husband will do good by his word and play the supporting role, etc. So beheno, to keep the mind calm and the body strong, here are the foods for this phase.

T3F1: Turmeric / Haldi

The West has discovered it too, the active curcumin compound in haldi has the ability to stop the degeneration of both the brain and the muscle and its antioxidant properties is the stuff that patent battles are made of. The turmeric in India is consumed both tender and mature, and in all its forms remains extremely useful. It is also being used for its ability to prevent eye strain, protect the heart, nerves and what have you, so don't miss out on this — but don't have it in a capsule form. It works best when it's part of a wholesome diet, so let's not turn into people who eat raw salads and pop turmeric pills. By the way, it's also an anti-depressant.

How to use it:

- In tadkas for dal / sabzi / khichdi. Follow the pattern taught at home about when exactly to add it while cooking.
- Tender turmeric — make a pickle or add in chai with lemongrass, ginger and honey.
- Add a pinch of turmeric to chana or masoor dal paste, mix it with milk and use it while bathing — especially useful to prevent pigmentation and lines post pregnancy.

T3F2: Moong — the Bean, Dal and Both Akha and Dhula

Amongst all the lentils, the most satvik bean is moong. If you have ever been to an ashram or on a yoga holiday, this is most likely the dal you ate. It remains the most precious dals in the eyes of our grandmoms for its easy digestibility, dense nutritional profile — folic acid, Vit B6, minerals, proteins, etc. — and for its neutral taste. Moong dal is the least gas-forming of all dals, a good quality to have if you are an expectant mother. Moreover, it helps you accelerate fat-burning, and reduces the risk of all degenerative diseases, including diabetes, BP and cancer.

How to use it:

- Sprout them overnight and cook them well for maximum nutrient absorption.
- Make dal or khichdi out of it.
- Make chatpata items like chivda or chilla out of it to kill the boredom of eating bland food without the risk of eating junk.

T3F3: Rice, Bhat, Chawal

You have waited for this one too. Hand-pounded, single-polished or just plain white rice and not the unpolished / brown versions. Eat your local rice, get it from the local markets and don't crib, please. If you can order nappies from Dubai and USA, then you or yours can surely make a trip to the local market too. Also, don't worry about the hundred opinions about rice. For starters, it's medium and not high on the glycaemic index. And then you will be mixing it with plant proteins like dals / lentils, and adding ghee — together this mixture or that of dahi-chawal or kadhi-chawal or even egg curry-rice or meat biryani is low on GI. Also, remember it has the resistant starch that helps the gut bacteria, and that this will be one of the first weaning foods for your baby. Spiritually, the grain of rice symbolizes health and growth, as well as the ability to let go and move on. Pretty much your go-to grain then.

How to use it:

- Cook rice and eat with dals / lentils / kadhi / dahi / milk.

- To make pej or kanji — a light soup that retains the Vit B of rice and is light to digest.

- Give a tadka or chokha to last night's leftover rice to turn into a quick and delicious breakfast meal.

The T3 Meal Plan

Timings	Meals	Notes
Meal 1 – On rising	Almonds and raisins – both soaked / or dry fruits and nuts / or fresh fruit	Choose one nut and complement it with a dry fruit: cashews and apricot / dates and walnuts / almond and raisins. A sweet and mineral-rich start to the day.
Meal 2 – Breakfast + Vit B complex / multivitamin / pregnancy vitamin	Any homemade nashta or jowar or ragi porridge (made at home)	Shift the first tea to 2 hours post rising.
Meal 3 – Mid-morning	Nariyal pani / kokum or nimbu sherbet / neera	Stay hydrated.
Meal 4 – Lunch + flaxseed or Omega-3, Vit B12	Roti + sabzi + tender turmeric achaar / or dal-rice / or khichdi / or dahi-rice + sprouted and cooked moong made in dry style.	Roti can be ragi or jowar or wheat. Rice can be alternated with foxtail millet too. Have raw turmeric achaar at least twice a week. Keep up with the 2 tsp of ghee.

Timings	Meals	Notes
Meal 5 – Mid-meal	Rawa-nariyal laddoo / peanut or rajgeera chiki / fresh seasonal fruit	If you have some special laddoo at home, have it here. Ensure that it has ghee and seeds like peanut or sesame that add to the essential fatty acid intake.
Meal 6 – Evening meal by 5 and 6 p.m.	Any homemade nashta item / homemade chivda with dahi / mathri with achaar / paneer toast / ragi dosa / fresh fruit milkshake	A wholesome meal. Don't drink chai / coffee after this. Your appetite will fluctuate, so eat according to hunger and don't stress over dinner, you can go for a very light dinner.
Meal 7 – Dinner + mixed carotene, Vit C	Rice kanji or pej with pinch of turmeric, hing and kalanamak. You can even add some dal ka pani if you like. Or dal-rice or khichdi or roti-sabzi-dal	Depending on how hungry you feel, pick the pej or the full-dinner options. Both are right and one is not better than the other, it is all dependent on your appetite.
Meal 8 – Bedtime + calcium citrate 1000mg	Haldi doodh – add sugar to taste	Continue to add jaiphal and cashews if sleep is an issue or you experience swelling in your feet or had a tiring day.

Important Notes for T3

· *Expect quite a bit of weight gain in this phase and that necessitates a bigger commitment towards both eating correct and exercising.*

· *If you are expecting swelling in your feet or lethargy in the evening, put your feet up as often as you can. Keep up with your yoga asanas.*

· *Keep up with eating local vegetables and the chutneys in the main meals as they lead to a slow steady rise in blood sugars and better energy levels through the day.*

· *Cut down on tea and coffee, especially the evening cups, as it will interfere with sleep at night.*

· *In the same vein, no late-night movies. Catch afternoon shows if you have to; carry a little snack and don't eat that stale theatre food.*

· *Pay special attention to hydration. Sugar and salt in packaged, processed foods, even if it's health food, will leave you dehydrated.*

· *Wear more open, breathable clothes to assist the thermo-regulation processes of the body.*

· *Continue avoiding places where you will be exposed to secondary smoke, sheesha or alcohol fumes.*

- *Take a Vit D supplement of 1000IU if you have an ache or pain in your legs or back.*

- *Feeling a bit tired or a bit heavy is pretty normal at this stage, so tweak your exercise intensity but do not give up on it. From Central Park in NYC to high Himalayan villages, women stay active and exercise even during T3, be it running or carrying a load of wood from the jungles. It's us urban women of developing countries who take it a little too easy or are simply scared of moving.*

- *If you find yourself involuntarily reaching under your t-shirt to scratch the stomach, then it's the first sign of blood sugars not stabilizing. Get moving, add ghee and other essential fats to your diet, soak, sprout and cook your legumes before you eat them, and don't forget to be a stickler to the bedtime routine.*

The NRI mommy

Timing	Meals – USA, UK, EU, NZ and Australia	Africa	UAE
On rising	Dry fruits or fresh fruit	Fresh fruit or nuts	Fruit or dates
Breakfast + Vit B or multivitamin	Egg and bread or cheese and bread or full fat / whole milk + fruit / ragi malt / millet porridge	Chapati and egg or poha or thepla	Egg and bread with halomi/ idli / poha
Mid-morning	Nimbu sherbet with kalanamak	Fresh fruit / sugarcane juice	Nimbu pani / kokum sherbet
Lunch + Vit B12 (especially Africa because of the heat), Add ghee to lunch and dinner	Beans and rice / lentil soup and bread / dal rice	Ugali – githeri Sukuma wiki / lentils and rice / sweet yam and dahi	Roti sabzi / hummus and pita with batata hara / rice and lentils
Mid-afternoon	Prunes or fresh fruit	Laddoo or local fruit	Olives or prunes

Timing	Meals – USA, UK, EU, NZ and Australia	Africa	UAE
Mid-evening	Cheese/ peanut butter/ avocado on toast or rice cracker + pumpkin/ melon seeds	Khakra with ghee or avocado on toast or boiled egg	Til or pista sweet or laddoo or cheese and bread
Dinner + Vit C, mixed carotene or antioxidant	Khichdi / pasta and veggies / daliya / rice pej	Teff bread or roti with veggies made in coconut curry or lentil soup or khichdi or dal-rice	Rice and lentils/ biryani and raita/ kebab and roti
Late night	Milk with nutmeg		

HERITAGE RECIPES FOR T3

Recipe 1: Lolo

Contributed by Simmi Harpa, Nagpur / Dubai

Rujuta says: The healthiest pancake, one that is just rightly spiced and will keep sugar cravings down.

Stepwise instructions:

- Heat a good amount of ghee in a pan. Add jaggery to it. Once the jaggery has melted and mixed, switch off the flame.
- Add this to whole wheat aata. Add jeera seeds to it.
- Make a tough dough and roll it into small but very thick rotis.
- Put on a tava on slow flame, and let it get crisp from inside. It takes 5-6 minutes for 1 lolo to be crispy and well-cooked from inside. Keep on applying pure ghee on tawa.

This lolo helped me maintain my sugar levels in the third trimester (gestational diabetes).

Recipe 2: Hardeli masala

Contributed by Prerana Pal Karmokar, Raipur, Chhattisgarh

Rujuta says: Garlic helps lactation and the other spices keep gas and flatulence down. Besides, it's great to taste.

Stepwise instructions:

- In a pan, heat ghee.
- Add crushed garlic and fry until golden brown.
- Add haldi, saunth and hing.
- Add salt to taste.
- Mix well and cool before eating.

This recipe is a wet paste that can be eaten with rice or chapati. It helps heal the body post-pregnancy and, during the last month of the third trimester, prepares the body to heal faster.

Recipe 3: Red rice porridge with green lentils

Contributed by Rajashri Vinod, Sharjah

Rujuta says: A good one for a Sunday or a holiday when you want to eat something nice but healthy.

Stepwise instructions:

1. Wash and soak rice and moong dal together for an hour with 3 cups of water.

2. Transfer the soaked rice and dal with water to the pressure cooker. Add methi seeds and garlic. Cook for 3 whistles. Turn off the heat.

3. Grind ½ cup of shredded coconut with ½ cup of water and squeeze thick milk from the coconut. (Add extra water to extract second milk and third milk for other dishes.)

4. When pressure drops, remove the weight and open the lid. Add salt, coconut milk, curry leaves.

This has helped me a lot in the last trimester. It helped in keeping up my strength and stamina, as well as eased fatigue before the delivery date.

Recipe 4: Batisa

Contributed by Shazia Deshmukh, Mumbai

Rujuta says: Stabilizes blood sugars and helps kick-start the day with high energy that won't slump in the afternoon

Stepwise instructions:

- Hand pound almonds and pista to a fine powder.

- Cut kharik (dry dates) and powder them.

- Fry goond (edible gum) in pure ghee till it is nice and fluffy.

- Grate the dry coconut finely.

- Mix all the ingredients in a bowl, add sugar and ghee and mix it by hand.

It is to be taken first thing in the morning, a spoonful with a glass of warm milk, right up to six months post-delivery.

Recipe 5: Bhoplyacha salanche chutney (Pumpkin skin dry chutney)

Contributed by Rujuta Diwekar

The perfect mix to soothe your intestines and add some spice and essential fats to your lunch and dinner. Works like magic on that sweet tooth.

Stepwise instructions:

Pumpkin is one of the most underrated vegetables.

Its versatility ensures that every region of India has a unique pumpkin preparation, right from petha to raita to subzi to thalipeeth. Like a true super food, every part of the pumpkin, from the peel to the seed, is used.

- Grate the pumpkin skin.

- In a kadhai, heat oil, add mustard seeds, asafoetida and turmeric powder. Add the grated skin and roast for a while.

- Add grated dry coconut and some til seeds and roast this mixture some more.

- Add salt.

This is a dry chutney and can be stored for a week.

Recipe 6: Mau bhat, Bhatachi pej (Rice gruel)

Contributed by Rujuta Diwekar

Again written for the husband; allows you to contribute, and for your wife to feel rejuvenated and rehydrated. Trust me, she will love you more after this.

Stepwise instructions:

- Take one measure of single-polished, hand-pounded rice (you should be able to find this online if not in your local kirana store).

- Add 7 measures of water and either pressure cook or cook on an open flame till the rice is completely cooked.

- Add a generous amount of ghee and some salt. (Tip: use non-iodized sea salt instead of table salt for a distinct flavour.)

- You can follow the above recipe for bhatachi pej or rice gruel. The only change you need to make is that instead of 7 measures of water, add 9-10 measures.

Note: This is also an excellent baby food. You can continue to give this to your children especially when they are sick. A great comfort food for adults too.

4

Post Pregnancy — A Return to Normal

Congratulations on the new arrival. In ancient times, and in not-so-ancient times, a safe delivery was considered a rebirth for women. And even though the evolution scales as well as our society are heavily tilted in favour of the baby, if we look hard enough, there are hidden / indirect practices to safeguard the health of the new mother.

My paternal grandfather lived in a big wada in Vasai, a small coastal town on the outskirts of Mumbai. The layout, with its big doors, high ceilings and the fact that it was large enough to have at least seven different families sharing space together, fascinated me. But what fascinated me more was the balantini chi kholi: the special room for the woman who had just delivered. It was a small room with no windows, and that is where the woman who had just given birth would stay for forty long days, almost like living in a cave. Cut off from the household and her official duties, as if being in a silence retreat, and on a satvic diet. And yet, if she did want to emerge from her cave, she could come out, soak up the sun, watch the other kids in the family play on the jhula and request for what she wanted from the kitchen.

Architecture is a wonderful thing because it documents our way of life, our priorities, and tells history better than any book. Women being cut off from outwardly sensory distractions would almost force their minds to focus on themselves, to acknowledge that here they are, and that they must not forget about their existence in this moment, only to be rudely reminded at menopause that they sacrificed their life for children. Essentially, a lesson delivered without uttering a word: women must realize that not looking after themselves doesn't turn them into better mothers.

And this ability to think about ourselves before the baby, like they tell us in the safety briefing during air travel, needs strength. This strength comes from the spine, the spine that has supported the womb, allowed the uterus to expand, and given the pelvis its flexibility. The next forty days are 'thank you, my friend' time. Feeding and lactating, carrying the baby around, changing nappies, everything from here on is also going to burden the spine. So the key here is to not just rebuild the strength in the spine but to also make it stronger than ever. Also, the undervalued aspect of getting back in shape is that it is the bone density and musculature around the spine that make it possible for you to flaunt that flat stomach and round butt.

But again, whether we stay there as unchallenged fitness queens or continue to make the one step forward and two steps backwards journey towards weight loss will depend entirely on our attitude. Whether we are sensible enough to be patient, and fearless enough to eat in such a way as to rebuild bone and muscle density, and support the fat-burning processes of the body.

If we take the impatient and insensible route of crash-dieting, then the body may lose weight for a short while and even look like it has shrunk, but then we will begin to suffer from sacro-obesity. That's the kind of obesity where the composition of the muscle cells, sarcomere, changes to accommodate more fat and less muscle protein.

So you might fit back into the same size of jeans, but they don't quite look the same on you. And now, because you are overall fatter than what you used to be, your vulnerability to developing lifestyle diseases like insulin resistance, diabetes, obesity itself increases.

There are women in their late fifties who tell me that they can't lose their stomach ever since they delivered their baby, who is probably now thirty! These conversations amused me to no end when I was younger, but the older I get I realize how easy it is for women to lose themselves in the act of raising a child. So let's look at how you can maintain a balance between looking after the child and yourself, without compromising on either.

FAQs for Post Pregnancy

1. How soon can I exercise post delivery?

The core principle of exercise is adaptation, which happens during rest. The benefits of a workout can only be seen on a well-rested and well-nourished body. And since delivering a child is a physiologically and psychologically draining task, it's best to take the first forty to forty-five days off from exercise. By that I don't mean bed rest — walk your baby around the house, stand often, do the small tasks yourself, but expect to feel more tired while doing 'less' in this period. A well-rested body responds beautifully to exercise and a tired body gets sick due to it. So walk this path carefully. Nurture the body a step at a time, back to its prime. In less than four months, you will be back to running on the treadmill and squatting under that rack of weight that you used to pre-pregnancy. But right now think of yourself as a wise warrior who knows when to retreat and when to attack the gym. So, like a pro-athlete, take the two months off so that you can come back to the game and give it your best shot. When you do go back to exercise, take it a step at a time, take it slow and allow yourself three to nine months (depending on exercise history or lack of it) to get into the groove of things. No rushing this, or it will come back to haunt you with a pulled muscle, or worse, some hormonal disorder. Read the Notes on Exercise and follow the exercise plan after this two-month period.

2. Do I really have to eat those laddoos?

Yes. Little bite sizes if you want, but know that it's way healthier than digging into chocolate or the ice cream tub that you will crave for in the middle of the night if you fall short of calories in the day. And, much more importantly, they are nutrient-rich with phytonutrients that help you bring the gut bacteria back to its prime, stabilize blood sugars, and work at secretly maintaining that skin tone and hair density too. What's not to love about the laddoo? I often feel that, given the right positioning and packaging, this could well be the next big Indian import after yoga. Also Baba Ramdev ji, if you do start a line of post-pregnancy foods, I will take a 10 per cent royalty. Itna toh bantay boss.

3. Will I need any lactation aids?

You will have no problems with lactation if you keep the positive nitrogen balance — this is what they mean when they say that lactating women have higher protein needs. The easy way to get there is to eat wholesome, sleep on time and stay happy. A large part of lactation is demand and supply, so have an old aunt or a family elder help you teach your baby to latch and suckle. It will take a couple of tries, but the baby will learn. Stay patient, and from there on, your prolactin and oxytocin will take over and do the rest. Eating right at this time will also teach your baby to not do natak over food as they get older. How well or badly the mother behaves when it comes to food right after a child is born has a strong link to whether or not he will be a 'fussy eater'. And kids pretty much learn everything from watching us and not from our speeches. Having said that, the next section covers top foods for post-pregnancy, including some excellent lactation aids.

4. If it's a caesarean, will my weight loss be slower?

No, natural or caesarean has a much bigger effect on

the baby than on you. So if you were the one who was going to be born, then you should hope to come out of the vaginal channel — that's a better route for your bone and muscle density and the gut bacteria. If you are giving birth, either way it's cool. If your caesarean was a last-minute thing, then it's not much of a problem, and if your doc advised you against a natural delivery (and assuming that she / he has your interest at heart), then it's mostly because you are starting from a bit of an unfit place. Either way, if you take it a step at a time and celebrate the changes in your body, then it's only a matter of whether you get in prime shape in two months or twelve months. So even if you had gestational diabetes or hypertension or twins, however precious your pregnancy, it won't take time to get back in shape. A year is hardly any time to get back in fab shape. What's more, it's irreversible and well worth the effort and time.

5. When will my bleeding post delivery stop?

It will typically go on for a week to ten days, and the foods that are recommended post delivery (next section) will not just assist in helping you clear out the womb but will also ensure that you don't get tired or bleed excessively. So think of it as a biggish period and nothing else.

6. If I stay up to feed my baby, will it affect my recovery?

To be honest, the irregularity will be a bit of a drain, and that's exactly why I emphasize so much on fitness even before getting pregnant and then throughout the pregnancy.

> Physical strength and stamina can do magical things to emotions, as well as amplify mental strength. This is an important aspect to remember, because drugs and technology can help you pop a child, but nothing other than self-reliance that comes out of sheer physical fitness will help you tide through the initial months.

The baby will not just stay up but may sometimes get colic or cranky, all regular stuff for which you will require some stamina, strength and flexibility, both in the mind and the body, to remember that this, too, shall pass.

This is also why you should clear out the logistical stuff with, foremost, your partner, and mother / mother-in-law or house help even before you pop. Have the strength to both receive help and to be grateful for it.

The one thing today that does wear out young mommies is checking emails, playing Candy Crush or updating statuses on fb while up in the night with the baby. Don't do that. Allow your HPT and PTA (Hypothalamus – Pituitary – Thyroid and Pituitary – Thyroid – Adrenals) to unwind; don't subject them to the light and the stimuli from your gadgets. The last thing you want is to wake up tired or bloated the next morning because of this distraction.

7. How soon can I go out?

As soon as you feel up to it. Typically, this does take about forty to forty-five days, and in many communities there is also a strict confinement period. But then, like my grandfather's large home, today the world is a woman's oyster. Her little cave could be her home or her bedroom, but if you think visiting a friend, family or even a café close by is going to help you unwind, please do so. The balantini chi kholi in my ancestral home was located in such a way as to get an almost panoramic view of what's happening. So the woman could take part without participating in the whole tamasha, watch like an outsider from the inside, be a part of the chaos without getting affected by it. Logistically, I would say don't go to places that are more than ten to fifteen minutes away from home, and go to tried-and-tested places with vibes that soothe you and where there is a guarantee that you will be well looked after.

8. When will my period start, when do things go back to normal / when do I go back to work?

This could range anywhere from three-four months post delivery to when you stop feeding. The food and the routine that you are on will help you adjust to the new normal and help you get to the earlier normal levels in no time. The key is to get there a day at a time, progressively, and not rush your way to normalcy. Women who are driven and look after themselves, are in that sense never off normal or away from work. So their work is already happening and they are back within days of delivery.

Also a short note here: if you are planning to quit after using your maternity leave, please be dignified and open about it right from the beginning. Because that just leaves a bad precedent for women who are looking forward to coming back to work in full swing, post delivery. It creates that discrimination for pregnant women where they get treated like time bombs that will suck out salary, maternity benefits and leave. After all, it's women who change the world, and we must create a better environment for all working women.

9. Will a belt help me get a flatter stomach? My grandmom suggests tying a saree around the waist.

I totally don't recommend wearing those tight belts around the waist. They almost suffocate you and make it hard for you to breathe. Instead, wear nice, stylish clothing and flaunt that paunch nicely. It's not going to be with you forever, and that little fat and bump around the stomach will disappear as it receives oxygen and blood circulation. You do that by not wearing anything too tight or fitting and also by staying active and exercising. And once again, exercise works on a rested and not on a tortured body or a stressed mind.

The saree, typically a red saree, wrapped around the waist works like a spinal support without suffocating the breath. The reason women wore this was to help the spinal muscles, which feel a little weak post delivery, and also to help regain a better sense of balance and stride.

It's like swaddling. For the longest time doctors told us not to wrap babies even when grandmoms would urge us to do so. I come from a large family, so I could wrap babies in malmal and carry them around with my palms for the right support from the time I was ten. Now in the West, you are taught to swaddle babies as part of prenatal classes. Research takes time but does catch up with age-old wisdom. So listen to your grandmom and remember the rule: D for dadi not doctor or dietician.

10. My hair: will it fall or grey post delivery?

No, pregnancy won't do anything terrible to your hair, but a weak thyroid brought about by not eating correctly before, during and after will. So buckle up, eat and know that the right food is the stepping stone towards great hair, skin and a thin waist.

11. Is breastfeeding really necessary?

Breast milk has the bacteria that is best suited for your baby. You may introduce diluted desi cow milk in a few months, so search for the right source already. The other options are rice kanji, ragi satva, sattu and very diluted dal-rice combos. Nothing other than making informed choices is necessary, so choose how you want to raise your kids.

> ## BREASTFEEDING IN THE HIMALAYA
>
> One of the best things about the Himalayan societies, again, is how their architecture tells the story. The temple is the centre of every little village and is often the largest and the best-looking structure, with a large indoor space and a very large well-maintained aangan. Whenever we are trekking and pass a village, we stop by the temple. If you reach in the middle of the day, every adult is out in the fields or the jungle but one or two women will be left behind with all the kids of the village. They often hang out in the temple and coolly breastfeed their own kids, neighbours'

kids, just every kid, while stroking their heads and not even once leaving your eyes as they chat with you. So if you ask these women, breastfeeding is very important. Important enough to bunk work and stay back in the temple. I always leave with a prayer that they don't lose this way of life, and I always hope that the goddess is listening even if her doors are closed.

Top Nine Foods for Post-Pregnancy (T4)

I would again like to reiterate that the reason why the women I work with look very thin post pregnancy is because they are very fit to begin with. Some of my clients have had their gynys telling them that if they hadn't themselves delivered the baby, they wouldn't believe that such a flat stomach was possible in just twelve to sixteen weeks. So if you are starting from another kind of baseline, or were unfit during pregnancy, then show the strength to be kind to the body. Take it a step at a time, and this pregnancy will be the best thing that has happened to you in terms of fitness and size.

So what are the foods that help then? Have a list of nine now instead of just three, lucky you! ;)

T4F1: Goond / Dinka / Edible Gum

The natural gum literally helps you keep it all together, both in your mind and in your body. From nourishing the brain, to helping digestion and even boosting the immune system, it does it all for you. It is even known for its abilities to stroke you back to your sexual vigour (including tightening the vagina), so it is an anti-ageing agent of sorts. Anything that improves sexual vigour is essentially stuff that will help you improve insulin sensitivity, so don't forget this goond.

How to use it:

- Most popular use is as a goond laddoo — best used in the first month post delivery.

- Soak in water and make a kheer with milk, kesar and sugar to taste — best for the second month after delivery.

- If both these don't interest you, make yourself a herbal chai with it.

T4F2: Ajwain / Carom seeds / Ova

Your grandma's go-to herb for all digestion issues has antifungal and antibacterial properties which help protect both you and your progeny.

> The disturbed sleep cycle that a baby causes disturbs the stomach too, bringing with it gas and acidity. There is almost nothing that can cure it as instantly and compassionately as ajwain can.

The reason why I say compassionately is because, unlike other digestive aids, this one won't come in the way of nutrient absorption and will help you with excretion of all that's holding you behind.

How to use it:

- Ajwain ka pani — probably amongst the most popular post-pregnancy drinks in our country.
- Mix ajwain in the dough with which you plan to make your chapati — ajwain paratha, as it's often called — or add it to your rice kanji along with ghee.

- Mix it in ghee or sesame oil and apply it to your scalp and stomach; it will help nourish your scalp and skin.

T4F3: Almonds / Mamara badam

First of all, pick the local badam, the one you get from Kashmir or Kinnaur, basically from the Indian Himalaya. The tocopherols and the other phytonutrients in the mamra bring the lustre back to your hair and the glow back to your face. Besides, the essential fatty acids help both the bone and muscle density, helping you smoothen out the uneven appearance of fat on the stomach, butt and thighs.

How to use it:

- Soak overnight, peel and eat a few as a morning snack or any time in the day.
- Use it to make halwas, barfis and laddoos.
- When someone you truly love comes over, chill with them over a cup of kawha made with kesar, cinnamon and almonds.

T4F4: Bajra

The pearl millet, as the West loves to call it, has all the minerals, fibre and amino acids that are required for an accelerated recovery post delivery. It is immuno boosting, ensuring that your heavy period doesn't leave you vulnerable to developing itches, discharges or infections. Besides, it provides a good support system to both the thyroid hormones and insulin. Always eat bajra with generous amounts of ghee.

How to use it:

- Bajra roti or bhakri, easily the best way to eat it.
- Bajra kheer or porridge, the easiest and the quickest breakfast for working women.
- Bajra kheechiya — for this you need to get hold of a Marwari or Gujarati neighbour / relative / friend's mom who will send these over to you. Don't forget the dollops of ghee.

T4F5: Saunf / Fennel

Everyone's favourite mouth freshener is actually nature's miracle worker, with its volatile oils and antioxidant properties. Loaded with vitamins and minerals, it is known for its ability to prevent irritable bowel syndrome and tumours, and even has cancer-protective properties. Marwaris will often have paan with some gulkand and saunf as part of the routine that they follow post pregnancy called japa. They have it for its abilities to restore full vaginal and reproductive health. Now Nestle is gunning for a patent on the fennel flower, but trust Marwari bahus to flush down all their native wisdom down their toilets. I work with all communities, but the community with the largest number of girls who flush the laddoos instead of eating them are the Madus. All in the fear of getting fat. But now you know how it plays itself out — sacro-obesity.

How to use it:

- Fennel chai or variyali pani — saunf seeds mixed with water. Add khadi shakkar to taste.

- A tsp of roasted seeds post a meal with a bit of jaggery — especially good for preventing bad breath.

- Use it as a garnish if eating a halwa, or have it as part of a paan.

T4F6: Sesame/ Til

My favourite seed, loaded with essential fats and great to taste, this is the backbone of every ancient culture and remains the biggest supporter of strength in the spine and mind. An appetite regulator, it helps you burn the stubborn fat and regulate the blood glucose response. Versatile in the number of ways it can be used, this is the secret formula to the Arabic woman's complexion and ageless skin.

How to use it:

- Til laddoos and chikis — easily the best mid-meals, and make for a great snack even once you are back to work life.
- Til chutney — to lift your spirits and the taste of otherwise bland food.
- Til oil — best applied to skin before having a bath. Helps restore the natural tone and complexion, fights pigmentation and pregnancy spots.

T4F7: Aliv

In my book, *Indian Superfoods*, I called it the beauty pill for its iron-rich properties and ability to keep your fatigue and irritability levels at bay. This red little seed, especially when soaked in coconut water, will ensure that you don't get drained out with the bleeding that follows post delivery, and that your mineral stores stay constantly replenished.

How to use it:

- The aliv laddoo made with coconut and jaggery is the best thing that happened to this world. And while dark chocolate is only good for the brains of guinea pigs, this one works wonders for the brains of real women like you and me.
- Soak the seeds and use it to make a kheer.
- Don't like anything sweet? Crush it with the sesame and have it like a chutney.

T4F8: Coconut

Mother Nature's own nourishing milk: rich in lauric acid, which protects you from all kinds of infections and illnesses, nurtures your nerves, and has a soothing effect on the mind. The essential fat brings both stamina in the muscles and density of the spine, besides boosting your body's effort to let go of excess fat stores. A very important but often overlooked lactating agent; can't afford to miss out on this one.

How to use it:

- Nariyal pani and malai as a mid-meal, hydrating snack.

- Fresh coconut for garnishing and making laddoos / barfis, or simply on its own.

- The dried coconut lends itself beautifully to both chutneys and kheer, and if you would like a quick snack, mix it with jaggery and have it as an afternoon snack to prevent the evening fatigue.

T4F9: Methi seeds

They have now earned the reputation of 'lactation medicine' in maternity hospitals in the USA. So if you delivered in that country, you would get an American passport for your baby and methi, no they call them fenugreek seeds, post delivery and you would hold them close to your heart, tears in your eyes and all. But if you are in India, you would struggle with basics, like getting the mother's maiden name on the birth certificate, and would be dismissing the gangs of wise women who would be gunning for you with their laddoos.

But that story apart, methi seeds help you rejuvenate, regulate blood sugars, support the thyroid glands, and make it easier for you to lactate. So bite in.

How to use it:

- Best eaten with other dense nutrients, so a laddoo that incorporates ghee, sugar, goond, coconut and methi dana works the best.

- Use it in tadka while making pumpkin ka sabzi or raita.

- Not interested in any of the above? Soak it in water and drink, but they go better when accompanied by essential fats.

The Post-Pregnancy Meal Plan

Timings	Meals	Notes
Meal 1 – On rising	Soaked almonds / dry fruits / fresh fruit and 1 tsp of warm ghee or *Goond laddoo made with coconut and methi seeds and ghee	If you have woken up any time after 3 a.m., have this meal and then go back to sleep. *If you have had an unusually long night.
Meal 2 – Breakfast + Vit B complex, Vit C	Bajra kheer with dollops of ghee or ajwain paratha / kulith paratha with ajwain / poha	Have a nap either before or after this meal based on your and your baby's routine.
Meal 3 – Mid-meal	Hot water with ajwain or fennel seeds / glass of milk with dry fruit (like masala milk) / fresh fruit	Pick on basis of appetite.
Meal 4 – Lunch + Alpha Lipoic Acid or Flaxseed, Vit D or pregnancy vitamin	Bajra roti with ghee + doodhi / pumpkin / gourd sabzi + moong dal + dry coconut chutney + dal or dahi (home-set) + saunf and jaggery to finish the meal	You can have ragi / foxtail / rice if you had bajra in the morning. Make sabzi in ghee if possible and til chutney is good too.

Timings	Meals	Notes
Meal 5 – Mid-meal	Goond laddoo or aliv laddoo or dry coconut, jaggery, saunf, dhania seeds and peanuts –just mixed and eaten together	A must-have meal, alternate them. If not here, can also have as mid-morning or first meal.
Meal 6 – Evening meal	Aliv laddoo or badam halwa or roti or khakra (homemade) or thepla with ajwain + til and coconut chutney	Pick the option based on what you feel like. A fresh seasonal fruit is a good option too.
Meal 7 – Dinner + antioxidant with selenium, zinc and chromium + mixed carotene	Moong dal khichdi or rice and kultih dal or rice pej with ghee, laddoo and milk or foxtail upma with veggies	Go as light or heavy depending on what nights are looking like. And expect almost daily variations in appetite, don't judge yourself. Just eat as per your need.
Meal 8 – Bedtime + calcium citrate 1000mg	Milk with haldi, pinch of dry ginger / nutmeg, soaked aliv seeds + sugar as needed or *dry fruit powder if needed	*Add the dry fruit powder if you prefer a little biggish meal or you ate too little for dinner and are now feeling hungry.

Important Notes for Post Pregnancy

- *While you will experience a fluctuating appetite throughout the pregnancy, it is post the delivery that it will really swing.*

- *At all times, eat to a point of feeling light and know that if yesterday you felt light after one bhakri, tomorrow you may feel light post two, and day after you may feel stuffed at half.*

- *You may experience swings only at one meal and the others may almost be in a steady state. Know that this is normal.*

- *Expect some aversions or nausea to certain meals on a day where you have had a compromised or disturbed sleep in the night.*

- *How quickly you lose weight post pregnancy and how well you lactate will depend on how well you recover. So take all the help you can and really don't sweat the small stuff.*

The thyroid gland works very hard, almost overtime, to help you with your pregnancy; it needs to be nurtured back to normalcy. If you cut down on calories right now, you are playing with your thyroid health and may land up with a post-pregnancy hypothyroid issue long term.

- When you roll laddoos, roll them into a small size so that you can have as many as you need at one time and the sight of a large one does not put you off.

- You can even just drink a cup of kulith (more watery than regular dal) with ghee and one tsp of cooked rice if you are coming down with a cough or infection.

- While a daily massage by midwives with the expertise is extremely useful, if you do not have access to one, massage your body with til oil and leave it on for fifteen to thirty minutes before having a bath.

- If you feel too tired or are unable to sleep in the night, massage the soles of your feet with ghee and apply coconut oil to your scalp.

HERITAGE RECIPES FOR POST-PREGNANCY

Recipe 1: Aliv laddoo (Halim, garden cress)

Contributed by Rekha Diwekar, Mumbai

Rujuta says: Easily my favourite and helps meet all post-natal nutrient needs. Make these for lactating woman you know. Essential for the microbiome too.

Stepwise instructions:

- Soak 50 gm of aliv in coconut water or in milk for an hour.

- Mix the aliv with freshly grated coconut. Add grated jaggery (roughly half the quantity of the grated coconut).

- In a brass vessel, heat a small quantity of ghee and then add the jaggery, coconut and soaked aliv seeds.

- Heat the mixture, stirring continuously till it gets cooked.

- Roll into laddoos.

Because of the use of fresh coconut in the recipe, these laddoos will not last longer than a week even in the refrigerator.

Recipe 2: Goond raab

Contributed by Sandhya Ranawat, Rajasthan / Singapore

Rujuta says: The brother or father can step in this time. You can make this for your sis / daughter instead of her mother doing it all the time. Barely takes any cooking at all, and you are intelligent enough to follow simple instructions in English.

Stepwise instructions:

- Heat up ghee in a heavy bottom pan.
- When hot enough, add goond (edible gum) and stir.
- It will puff up slowly. Once puffed up properly (it takes less than 2 minutes), add hot water.
- Stir it till the goond dissolves completely.
- Add jaggery, saunth, piparamul, almonds and coconut.
- Let it boil for 2 minutes. Serve hot.

Raab provides vital energy and strengthens the backbone. Given on the second / third day post-delivery.

Recipe 3: Methi seed usal

Contributed by Aarati Marathe, Pune

Rujuta says: Fenugreek is great for recovery and lactation. Sprouting it makes it even easier for the body to assimilate nutrients.

Stepwise instructions:

- Soak the methi seeds overnight.

- Drain the water the next day, dry the seeds with a dry cotton cloth and tie the seeds in the same cloth to get the sprouts.

- Heat the oil, add mustard, cumin seeds, asafoetida, curry leaves and turmeric powder.

- Add methi sprouts. Stir fry and close it with a lid.

- After one steam, add kokum, little bit of chilli powder and salt. Add some water and cook for some time.

- After the seeds are half cooked, add jaggery and cook for a little time.

- Garnish it with coconut and coriander.

- Serve with roti / bhakri.

Recipe 4: Hareera

Contributed by Arti Gautam, UP

Rujuta says: The hair-skin-nails formula that your grandmom approves of.

Stepwise instructions:

- Grind coarsely 1 cup dry dates (chhuhara), ½ cup almonds, ½ cup cashews, ¼ cup walnuts

- Heat 4-5 tbsp ghee in a pan, add 1 tsp carom seeds (ajwain) when hot. Add ground mixture of nuts when it splutters.

- Roast the mixture on a low flame till it becomes aromatic.

- Add 2½ to 3 cups of water and let it boil.

- Add 1 tsp of dry ginger powder, ¼ tsp of cumin seeds, a handful of raisins and jaggery powder to taste. Let it simmer till the ghee starts separating.

- Finally finish it with 1 tbsp ghee.

- Let it cool and store it. Can be stored for 2-3 days.

Good for lactation and energy.

Recipe 5: Coconut-poppy seeds kheer

Contributed by Uma Kulkarni, Maharashtra

Rujuta says: It can be your go-to meal on late or tiring nights; it aids recovery and enhances sleep quality too.

Stepwise instructions:

- Roast a cup of grated dry coconut.

- Roast a tablespoon of poppy seeds (khus khus) till fragrant.

- Grind both of these in a jar till it has a grainy consistency.

- Bring 3 cups of milk to boil.

- Mix the coconut-poppy seeds mixture well and let it simmer for another 5 minutes.

- Add a pinch of cardamom powder, a pinch of grated nutmeg and 4-5 almonds that are soaked, peeled and cut. Add sugar to taste.

If the baby is breastfed, this recipe will definitely make him sleep for longer hours at a stretch.

Recipe 6: Kalo jeera rosun bhaja

Contributed by Debasree, Kolkata

Rujuta says: A mixture of spices that help in digestion and aid lactation. Especially good if you are feeling bloated.

Stepwise instructions:

- In a tadka pan, add ghee, jeera, kalonji (onion

seeds), ajwain, 2 to 3 cloves of garlic, a pinch of black pepper.

- Lightly fry and then add rock salt.
- Pour on a little rice (2 to 3 morsels); rest of the rice can be eaten with usual curries, etc.

This is a popular thing we eat in the beginning of our meal (lunch) post-delivery. My mom told me that it helps in contracting the uterus, is anti-infection and helps in digestion.

Recipe 7: *Balantini chi sol kadi*

Contributed by: Medini Pathare Korgaonkar, Goa

Rujuta says: Kokum is a super food for more reasons than one and along with coconut, it will also pave the way for you to get your sex drive on the upswing again.

Stepwise instructions:

- Soak a few kokum pieces in water (add just enough water for the kokum pieces to swim in it) for an hour or two. This helps the kokum to release its juice.
- Add some sugar and salt.

- As you start setting your table for the meals, grind some freshly scraped coconut with 1 or 2 cloves of garlic, ova (ajwain) and a pinch of Kashmiri red chilli for colour (we use small red chillies from Goa). Strain the juice and add it to the kokum juice.

- Finally, decorate with finely chopped coriander. Add sugar and salt as per your taste.

It's a very good digestive and deworms your system.

Recipe 8: Melogra

Contributed by Roopa Vasan, Bangalore

Rujuta says: Dill or shepu is the secret here, cleverly blended with lentils and rice, it's the perfect combo for mineral and micro-nutrient assimilation.

Stepwise instructions:

- Boil toor dal along with dill leaves together with a pinch of turmeric and some oil. Give about 6 whistles in the pressure cooker.

- Make a paste of coconut (1 small bowl), rice flour (2 tsp), green chilli (1), coriander leaves, turmeric (¼ tsp), hing (a little), garlic (1 or 2 small pods) and blend them into a smooth paste.

- Mix this paste along with the dal and dill leaves and allow this mixture to boil on a low flame for 10 minutes. Add water if needed as per the consistency you want.

- Add some mustard seeds tadka at the end.

- Serve hot with rice and ghee.

Recipe 9: *Manathakkali vathals*

Contributed by Shreekala Ganesh, Kerala / Tamil Nadu

Rujuta says: Simple, easy and the drumstick or the moringa leaves are already in the news for being nature's very own pharmacy. Though local berries or moringa remain undervalued and poor man's food in our country.

Stepwise instructions:

- Roast sundried manathakkali vathals (a particular type of berry found in Kerala and Tamil Nadu) in ghee and eat it with cooked rice.

- Also, leaves of the drumstick plant can be roasted this way and can be had with rice.

Boosts milk production in new mothers.

Recipe 10: Ajwain pani

Contributed by: Sarika Dhiraj Ostwal, Vansda (near Surat)

Rujuta says: One more for the husband, not that I have a problem if you can do more. But the ones I have marked are compulsory ;).

Stepwise instructions:
- Add 3 tsp of ghee in a pan and heat it.
- Add 3 tsps of gud (jaggery).
- Add 1 glass of water.
- After the gud melts, add 2 tsp of aajma powder (ajwain, carom).
- Let it boil and then serve hot.

It's very good for the first three days post delivery to remove all the waste from the body. After three days of liquid aajma you can start aajmo (in solid form) with badam, khobra, dink, kharik and gud.

Notes on Exercise

... to Do or Not to Do?

That is not the question. The question truly is: how do you plan to equip yourself with the new role of motherhood? Where will you possibly derive the strength and the endurance from? It's a job of a lifetime and both the brain and the muscles must be well equipped to take it, shall I say, head on.

While exercise helps with strength, endurance, flexibility and reflexes, the one that is of paramount importance during and after pregnancy is strength. The three main reasons are:

1. Better strength means a toned body. Improved muscle tone means higher insulin sensitivity, so

less chance of diabetes or other complications during pregnancy.

2. Has a protective effect on the weight-bearing joints — hip and spine — as they are prone to hyper flexibility during pregnancy.

3. A stronger body, especially spine, also means a faster return to a flatter stomach post pregnancy.

> The one exercise that dramatically improves the strength of the muscles and lowers the total body fat is strength training. And it is exactly this exercise that is avoided either out of the fear that it will make us very bulky or some random safety concern that lifting weights is not very conducive for pregnancy.

Readers of *Don't Lose Out, Work Out* know the whole funda behind strength training, but just to remind everyone else — heavy lifting is what pregnancy is all about. Strength training, on the other hand, is about training light, light enough to perform twelve to fifteen reps with good form. It costs less than thirty minutes per session, it doesn't disturb your blow-dried hair, and it improves blood circulation and oxygenation to your ovaries. I mean, if you are weight training, always have safe sex coz the ovaries are always ready, you know what I mean ;).

Even during pregnancy, it's a safe exercise to perform because it's a non-impact exercise. You can use machines that allow you to train specific muscle groups without overloading or stressing your core or your baby. One of the reasons why you are not asked to jump during pregnancy is that it is an impact exercise, but that's not the case with strength training. Also, post pregnancy, the lax muscles will get back to a better tone once you introduce the stimuli of weight / strength training.

But does that mean you can't do cardio or yoga, and what about bed rest? Answers below under the FAQs section.

But before we go there, there are two important concepts you need to understand about exercise during and after pregnancy:

1. *Exercise and the gut bacteria*

Amongst the many unknown benefits of exercise is its effect on the microbiome. The microbiome plays such a huge role in a healthy pregnancy, and later even in the health and well-being of your baby, that compared to this the benefits of fat loss or a flat stomach pale in comparison. Exercise specifically increases the strength of butyrate-producing bacteria and thus helps you alleviate not just the problems of constipation and gas but also of insulin resistance and immune function. In fact, exercise is so critical for good health that if you do have a doctor who has a very orthodox, rigid view about exercise, change the doctor.

> And here's another reason why you must make exercise a non-negotiable aspect of your life, not just for the muscles but also for the brain. The gut microbiota and the brain are closely linked, so exercise before getting pregnant to not be affected by stress; during, to not lose patience; and after, to not feel like a wreck.

You would need that dose of exercise, as the support it provides to the microbiota is an important preventive strategy for postpartum depression too.

2. Thermo-regulation

When we perform any exercise, the energy expenditure is broadly classified into two heads: i) the actual mechanical cost to the body, i.e. calories burned to perform that activity and ii) the calories burned to bring down the core body temperature.

During pregnancy, sometimes the calories required to bring down the core body temperature may dramatically rise, leading you to believe that you actually did something very heavy or strenuous to get this tired. But in reality, the tiredness could just come out of the energy spent to bring down / normalize the core body temperature that rises due to exercise. And that's why indoor workouts in well-ventilated spaces, breathable workout wear and hydration levels are of paramount importance in this phase of your life. They allow you to mechanically exert your strength and stamina while protecting you from feeling washed-out or tired.

FAQs for Exercise During and After Pregnancy

1. Can I do cardio during pregnancy?

For cardio or endurance / stamina exercises, it's better to cycle or swim as neither require you to carry your weight. That way not just the hip, back, knee and ankle, but even the womb and the baby are safe. You exclusively train the heart and lungs, receive the benefits of fat-burning and better blood circulation but rule out the risk of causing any stress to the core.

While walking is a safe activity to do, if you perform it as an exercise — as in, increase the challenge: walk uphill, briskly or do it for a fixed amount of time like thirty minutes etc., ensure that you are not a first-timer to exercise. Walk around all you want, but it is only safe as a form of exercise for people who are already fit. Read this part again.

> Walking is a weight-bearing exercise, something that loads your core — hips, back and abs — and if you are having a tough pregnancy and are asked to avoid heavy exercise, avoid walking and instead

choose the safe, non weight-bearing option of cycling or swimming, and of course, strength training.

Walking is more accessible than cycling or swimming but if safety is a concern, choose the latter. I really like indoor cycling as it's not just non-weight-bearing but also, with the AC and all, you can control the temperature and not sweat like a pig just because you worked out.

2. What about yoga?

It's a beautiful way of life and much more than exercise. And though it's largely considered safe to do once you are pregnant, it's best to go to a damn good teacher and study under her. Once again, I would recommend everyone read and follow the guidelines from *Iyengar Yoga for Motherhood*. I do hope specialized Iyengar yoga pregnancy classes become available online so people who are out of Mumbai can benefit. The classes typically start from the fifth month and there is a well-structured routine that is followed according to the month of the pregnancy. This allows both the woman and her baby to safely reap the benefits of better nutrient and blood supply while taking the stress off the weight-bearing joints.

3. What about Zumba / dancing / aqua yoga?

If you are already doing Zumba and dancing, then all you have to do is share the pregnancy news, expect a hug and a scream (Zumba and dance teachers are usually much more expressive than regular trainers). And then of course, instructions on what part of the class you can do and what you must avoid. Anything that leads to an impact or stresses the weight-bearing joints like spot running, jumps, etc., are best avoided. During the latter half of your pregnancy, sliding movements may get tougher for the ligaments of the knee. A well-experienced trainer can help tailor movements for you and the baby.

Aqua yoga or exercise, on the other hand, is no issue at all, since under water you are almost weightless. It's an excellent form of exercise for all those who have been advised bed rest, as being under water puts much less load on your body than even lying on a bed. And it allows you to strengthen the bones and muscle tone without causing any soreness. The eccentric movement, the one where your body has to contract with gravity or where muscles lengthen as a form of contraction, is absent in these forms of exercise, making it safe and injury-free for pregnant women. This is also one of the major fundas behind water births, which are considered least stressful for the baby.

4. My doctor has strictly advised against any form of exercise except for a walk. What now?

Gynaecs, orthos, heart surgeons, basically any kind of doctor, do not have training in exercise physiology, biomechanics, kinesiology, ergonomics, etc. And hence the misguided advice. There's tons on this subject in *Don't Lose Out, Work Out,* but here are the basics that you should be aware of:

- Exercise is critical for good health, a smooth pregnancy and delivery and a return to good body composition post delivery.
- Exercise is not just safe but recommended by all the gyny and obstetrician institutions of

the world, including the American College of Obstetricians and Gynaecologists.

- Any woman who can walk as a form of exercise (bear the biomechanical forces on her weight-bearing joints) during pregnancy, is fit enough to do yoga, weight training, cycling, swimming. In fact, of all these, walking is the most stressful on the joints.

- Fitness is specific in the pathways it employs, so while walking is great as a means of activity, it is strength training, swimming, yoga that will specifically work at improving strength, stamina and balancing abilities of the body. And at the same time, it will help improve glucose uptake and reduce chances of developing diabetes and hypertension during pregnancy, and post-delivery thyroid issues.

THE SQUATTING DELIVERY

I ran a gym in Ruia College, Mumbai, from 2005 to 2009. We had three gynys amongst our first ten

---

members. And as they discovered the benefits of exercise themselves, they began recommending strength training to women with PCOD. One of them would even deliver babies with the women in the squatting position, if they had the strength and endurance for it. The gravitational force is like a natural epidural, making labour and pushing the baby less stressful than the lying down position. In fact, yoga even has a name for it, kalika-asana, where the woman assumes a half-squat pose while delivering. And trust me, this is gonna come back, just like the good old Asian pot is making millions in the form of squatty potty.

5. The best time to exercise?

Any time is the best time as far as exercise is concerned, but during pregnancy, it's best to exercise post a meal, and evening is better instead of mornings. The very obvious reason is morning sickness, and you feel better in the latter half of the day, but there's more. Evening workouts ensure that you are not running out of energy for your daily tasks just because you exercised. And also that you are actually feeling fit enough to exercise and not just pushing yourself into doing it out of sheer willpower. This is because exercise in the evening is only possible if you have made the effort to eat right and stay well hydrated through the day. Remember, forced exercise has a detrimental effect on the gut microbiome. Matlab, no points for willpower during pregnancy; it's killing the main benefit you are hoping to achieve through exercise. Some other benefits of evening workouts:

- Evenings are cooler so less stressful for the body to lower the core body temperature during and post exercise. So you can work out more without getting tired.
- Allows for better assimilation of nutrients from dinner.
- Promotes good sleep.
- Improves chances of waking up fresh and energetic the next morning.

6. I don't have the energy to exercise.

No problem, take it easy. Go for a light stroll, watch kids playing in a park or squabbling over a game of football. Focus on eating better, staying hydrated and getting a good rest in the afternoon and nights. This will ensure that you will be up to exercise soon enough. You don't have to start with twenty or thirty minutes. Start slow, start small — five minutes a day — and build it up over a period of time, but keep the stimuli going. The thing with energy is that it increases when it is expended, so you have to break that cycle wisely. Also, if you exercise post a meal or after a fresh fruit, you are more likely to feel up to it. All the best.

7. Can I return to HIIT or functional training after delivery?

If you are not ten-fifteen years into HIIT or functional training, take a break and stick to the more traditional weight training or strength training exercises. Again, it's all about impact, and the less the impact and the more regulated the rest between the sets, the better for the body, especially for its thermo-regulation abilities. During pregnancy, use the machines that allow you to train muscles like the pecs (chest), lats (back), quads and hamstrings (legs), without the need to carry the entire body weight or strain the weight-bearing joints. Gyms today have biomechanically sound equipment with detailed instructions on how to use that info, and it's totally worth investing time and money in a good gym and a good trainer if you lack the confidence to do it on your own.

- Remember to stay active, walk around through the day.
- On a day you don't feel like it, skip the exercise even if it's your day to work out as per schedule.
- Work out at an intensity that you are comfortable with.
- Keep the duration to thirty to forty minutes, unless you are at an advanced level.

Weekly Training Calendar and Exercise Plan

1. Weekly training calendar during pregnancy and post delivery (after forty days)

Beginners (never worked out or less than 1 year)	Intermediate (1-5 years of some exercise or the other)	Advanced (5 and more and an active life)
Day 1 (D1) – Yoga	D1 – Yoga	D1 – Yoga
D2 – Rest	D2 – Cardio 20 mins	D2 – Cardio 20 mins
D3 – Weight training	D3 – Rest	D3 – Weight training
D4 – Rest	D4 – Weight training	D4 – Rest
D5 – Yoga	D5 – Yoga / rest	D5 – Yoga
D6 – Rest	D6 – Rest	D6 – Weight training
D7 – Rest	D7 – Weight training	D7 – Cardio 20 mins / rest / yoga

2. Safe and recommended weight-training exercises during pregnancy.

Target body part	Exercise name and a special tip	Advantages
Legs The largest muscle group that will bear all the weight you will gain during pregnancy. 1-2 sets with 10-15 reps each. Pick 2-3 exercises from the list.	Squats - Use your body weight or squat under a light bar. Leg extension - The seated extension machine. Seated leg curl - Avoid the one where you lie down on your stomach. Stiff leg deadlift - Only if you are used to it.	- Calf cramps, swollen feet and hypertension, each one of them can be prevented by training your legs smartly. - The key is to build stronger muscles and to provide the stimuli for accumulating more bone mineral density during and after pregnancy.

Target body part	Exercise name and a special tip	Advantages
Back		
An untrained back will bring with it a collapsed chest and sagging boobs. As the breast tissue enlarges, it's these muscles that literally form their back support and help them stay taut and firm. 1-2 sets with 10-15 reps each. Pick 2 exercises from the list.	Lat pull down - Use the machine and have someone bring the bar down to your shoulder height before you start. Seated rows - Use machines that don't squeeze your front body or learn to readjust distance from the chest pad. Shrugs - Use dumbbells for your shrugs and squeeze all the way to your ears.	- A toned back is a priceless asset during and post pregnancy. It ensures that you never have a bad back day, makes it easier for you to bear labour pain, and it is your secret route to getting back to a flat stomach post delivery. - A strong back also ensures that you don't get the duck walk during the last stages of pregnancy.

Target body part	Exercise name and a special tip	Advantages
Chest Chest is a pushing muscle and upper body strength is important to push the baby out. A stronger chest also ensures that your upper body stays upright and doesn't begin to collapse on the lower body. 1-2 sets with 10-15 reps each. Perform any 2 exercises.	Chest press - If you have never weight trained, use the machine. If you are a regular, continue with the dumbbell presses on the bench and always come up from one side. The bench / dumbbell press has at least 3 versions. Pec dec - Do them seated on a machine or use a cable cross over to do your flyes based on how regular you are in the gym.	- Your pectorals (chest muscles) play a big role in breast feeding, actually in how tired you feel while you feed. The stronger the chest, the happier you feel post the feed, the easier it is to cuddle her in your arms while she suckles away. - A lot of feelings of tiredness and fatigue come from the chest collapsing and the lungs not getting the full scope to breathe and oxygenate the entire system.

Target body part	Exercise name and a special tip	Advantages
Shoulders Toned shoulders help give you that petite appearance and ensures that only the bump shows and the rest of the body looks in great shape. 1 set each with 10–15 reps. Pick any 2 exercises	Overhead presses - Avoid if you have neck pain or a tendency to have swollen feet or BP issues. Side laterals - Sit or stand and use dumbbells; learn the right form. Rev flyes - Only if you have been used to it or the muscles get used while training the back too.	- Toned deltoids (shoulder muscles) sure look good but come to good use when you are carrying around your baby, burping her and carrying around a bag with all her stuff. - Also prevents frozen shoulder in the long run.
Arms These tiny muscles should be trained in proportion to the rest of the body. 1 set each with 10–15 reps. Pick any 2 exercises.	Dumbbell curl - Sit or stand while you do it. Dumbbell extension – Again, avoid if you have neck pain.	- Training the back and chest, uses these muscles. So if you are short on time, skip this. - Toned arms make your arms look longer and tauter.

Note:

- Weight train 1-2 times a week but never on back to back days.
- Limit the total number of sets to 12 per workout session.
- Ensure that you have had a meal before exercising or eat a fresh fruit before exercise.
- Carry a water bottle to sip on while working out.
- Eat a banana post exercise, before you leave from the gym.
- If you are feeling sick or had a late night, avoid exercise on that day.
- Take adequate but measured rests between sets.
- Please ensure that there is a proper warm up and cool down and include stretching in both.

Notes on Sleep

For all the talk on exercise and food, whether the two will really bear results, or scientifically speaking, the adaptation response of better fat-burning, bone density and inner peace, will depend on how much rest and recovery you can provide to the body. Pregnancy can be classified as a huge surge and then an equally sharp drop in some of the most anabolic hormones of the body — HGH, insulin and thyroid, to name a few. And it's good sleep that sets in the adaptation response, allows for the growth of the foetus, and turns this hormonally turbulent time into a smooth ride for you.

Maneka Gandhi, too, seems to understand the importance of sleep and hormones, and that's how we have the Maternity Bill. A landmark one, in which you have six months' paid leave from work. Sleep deprivation can play havoc on both our mind and body, and therefore it's used as an interrogation or even torture technique in the West, or at least that's what I saw in the TV series *Homeland*. It's easier to break people's resolve post a few nights of no sleep, even if it's simply a resolve to eat right, stay active and get some exercise. Turning us into anxious and moody moms instead of the yummy version we want to become.

Sleep, like all things in life, is affected by lifestyle factors of diet and exercise, and here's looking at the stuff that matters.

1. ***Food:*** Well, what can I possibly say about how food affects sleep and therefore, our well-being. We know this right from the time of the *Mahabharata*; one of Krishna's greatest life lessons is that one who eats too much or too little, sleeps too much or too little, is incapable of yoga. Yoga is that sense of union, whether it's with your baby, or simply your own self, and no wonder that women who are sleep deprived (or are overdoing it) don't feel like themselves or lose that union with themselves. Here are a few hacks that help:

- *Addition of ghee, coconut, white butter and other essential fats in the diet — for insulin.* Besides lowering the glycaemic index of the meals and ensuring that blood sugars stay steady post meal, addition of fat increases the satiety value of a meal. Which means that you actually feel fuller with a smaller amount, leading to a lowered caloric load and better assimilation of nutrients from every meal.

- *Addition of pulses in the diet — for leptin and GH.*

Whether in the form of dals, chillas or halwas and laddoos, pulses have a nutrient profile that, besides providing the body with amino acids and minerals, also help improve leptin sensitivity. Leptin is a hormone that tells the body when to stop eating, reduces midnight cravings and, much more importantly, calms the body down and closes the excretory responses of the body. This in turn helps your growth hormone function properly. That way you can actually sleep through the night and not wake up every now and then for sussu or hungry for some food.

- *The cashew milk nightcap — for the thyroid.*

Soak a handful of cashews in milk for a couple of hours, grind them, add more milk, and drink just before you go to bed. Works beautifully, almost like a drug, and without any side effects.

But with the rider that you have been eating right through the day. Great for the absorption of fat-soluble vitamins like A, E, D and K. Especially for Vit D, as it plays a role in sleep regulation, hormonal balance and boosting the immunity response of both the mother and the child. The effectiveness of vaccinations is also dependent on Vit D status, so it's important that you have enough to pass on to your child.

- *No gadgets while eating and feeding.*

While the above three help restore the hormonal balance, ensure accelerated fat-burning and boost the health of the skin and hair, using the phone while you are eating or while feeding the baby just kills it. The light emissions and the waves do come in the way of the HPA and

HPO axis (Hypothalamus – Pituitary – Adrenal / Ovaries), and will leave you bloated, agitated and sleep deprived. As we age, it's important to learn to be in the company of ourselves, to embark on the journey of figuring who we really are, and the phone really comes in the way of that too. Also, don't post pix of your baby bump while pregnant and cute pix of your baby post delivery on WhatsApp groups; it's kind of needy to be doing that and keeps you glued to the phone, refreshing feed all the time. People who are interested in you and the baby will visit you anyway, and the ones who are clapping or liking are just doing it for the heck of it. And early in your life, learn that claps or appreciation of baby pix is not for you. The baby is not your passport to love, appreciation and fondness from the family, colleagues or the rest of the world, so keep up with your own life anyway. And gain all that yourself, or it's too much pressure on the poor kid already.

- *Midnight meals.* If you do wake up in the middle of the night while pregnant or early in the morning post delivery, milk is a good meal to have. Have it the way you like it. You can even have homemade laddoos that are rich in essential fats so that your digestive system is not too stressed. And if you wake up to a nightmare, it's just acidity acting up, so a glass of milk with a tsp of cooked rice should do the trick. And don't forget that massage to the soles of the feet with kokum butter (see box on page 202).

2. *Exercise*: The big hormone regulator and stress-reliever, it plays a high value and underrated role in managing your sleep cycle. Regular exercise ensures that ovaries are well nourished, the muscles are toned and fat metabolism is at its optimum. It is specifically important for the big three — insulin, growth hormone and thyroid — and ensures that they stay in a balanced state, promoting good sleep and a sense of well-being. A well-rested body produces anti-inflammatory adipokines (hormones that fat cells secrete), while in a sleep-deprived state the same fat cells will produce inflammatory adipokines (leading to swelling, bloating and even illness). So if you want to avoid swollen feet and face while pregnant, or a bloated stomach post pregnancy, exercise is non-negotiable and will actually train your fat cells to

function optimally. The exception of forty days post delivery still stays, and know that activity is still safe during this period. Walk around with your baby; just don't stress the body.

3. ***Room temperature and clothes:*** Most wives crib about how the fat or hormone-insulated husband turns the bedroom into an icy torture chamber. Well, with pregnancy the tables have officially turned. Pregnancy is an overheated state, so take charge of the remote and set it at a temperature that you are comfy with. Use the timer, AC and fan, window and fan, whatever it takes to ensure that you are not going through night sweats or anything that could wake you up. Throw the husband out of the bedroom if he complains or teach him to take a leaf out of your book and sleep with extra chaddars. All you want is to sleep peacefully and have the fat cells produce anti-inflammatory adipokines.

Clothes — breathable wear at all times, but when you are sleeping, minimally clothed or wear nothing at all. Helps not just with temperature regulation but even dries out the yeast infection in the vagina and other harmful bacteria and promotes growth of good bacteria. The gut bacteria is also a sleep booster, in fact, plays a role in Vit D assimilation too, which further plays a role in sleep regulation. So take off and sleep off, Princess; the good bacteria, and not the frog, awaits you.

4. ***Afternoon nap and recovery***: While night sleep is extremely important for recovery both during and post pregnancy, the afternoon nap is also crucial. The game-changer in pregnancy are the hormones, and for them to function at the optimum, rest, food, exercise and lifestyle must be well regulated.

> From the day you know you are pregnant, work at getting an afternoon nap, and continue till you are feeding. It's not about sleeping for hours together in the afternoon, but catching those forty winks post lunch, a quick ten-twenty minute nap will do it.

In fact, an Arabic proverb says that one who naps post lunch and strolls post dinner never needs to see a doctor. Stroll, not a brisk walk; it's that balance between activity and rest that leads us to a good life. The nap is called beauty sleep for the same reason: it regulates hormones and so prevents pigmentation and hair loss. The daily massage right after delivery is also another way to promote rest and recovery; rather, it puts them in the forefront of a young mother's life.

THE KOKUM BUTTER SPA

The secret to a good restorative sleep, especially in the late pregnancy phase, is to massage the soles of your feet with kokum butter. If you live in Maharashtra, you will get it for less than forty bucks at any of the Malwani melas, and if you don't live there, don't crib, pick it up from Goa on your next trip there, and post this book, you will even find it online. The thing with these effective remedies is that they are local and not packaged to attract the attention of the young buyer; they are so native that they won't even make it to your farmer's market, which by the way, is selling broccoli, avocado and kale, for heaven's sake. See, India's economy is on an upswing, so time is ripe now to gain some confidence and invest interest in the native produce, right? That way you would have introduced your daughter to kokum butter even before she was born and not waited for her to discover it when she was on a trip to China (ya, I think tourism to London, Paris is likely to fall by the time she's vacationing alone).

So how it works is that it helps reduce the vata (gas and bloating-related ailments which include disturbed or broken sleep and acidity) element of the body. If you are the conscious type, rub the kokum butter to your feet when you are alone because you are likely to burp or fart right after that. Other alternatives are ghee or coconut oil, and obviously just sleep post this: don't walk around right after that and risk slipping. It's totally safe to walk on waking up though, as the body would have absorbed it all by then. Don't like massaging the feet? Try the medicated nasal ghee drops that some gaushalas sell; again, a compassionate and kind way to put your body to sleep.

Ancient cultures talk of lifestyle correction to avoid doctors or medicine while the modern lifestyle promotes consumerism or a singular remedy like an apple to keep the doctor away. The latter never works and the former takes a lot of work.

An Afterword

'This is a moment we will remember together, forever,' said Saif about the moment when Taimur was born and he first met Kareena's eyes. And however true that may be, moments get over and life takes over. Oh! He cries when I sit and smiles when I walk. Oops! She's colicky today. Why won't he sleep? Is she still hungry? Our children come into our life and everything from that moment changes. At least, our priorities do, and so does our waistline and even the bottom line. The bottom line, I am guessing, you have long-term plans for and is all sorted. The waistline, I hope this book helps you get one that is smaller than you have ever flaunted.

But then there is another line. The line that we often cross. The one between love and attachment. While love for our child liberates us from all bondages and changes the way we view the world and its happenings, our attachments make us feel constantly concerned, scrutinized and the world seems to be against us. There is a system, almost from the doctor to the tailor, to make us feel inadequate; you are not lactating enough, you are not feeding enough, you are not being a good mother in general! Almost all my clients have voiced this complaint in one way or the other. The charms of having the baby, the reward almost, never dies, they always remain a source of inspiration, joy and fulfilment. But Hindu or Muslim, rich or poor, right or left, the one thing that we obsess with — is my child eating enough? Will she get taller or fatter than me? What should I give her after I stop feeding? Rice pej? Ragi kheer? Sattu or formula? Is it okay to have milk?

And then school? Never finishes her dabba! Always eats in front of other people and is fussy around me. Uses food to blackmail me into video time. Gets sick after eating out, can barely tolerate spices. Can

I give him sugar? What's the right age to introduce it? And when she hits teenage, what can I do about her iron?

The questions about child's nutrition are endless and we will fuss over them till we die. And hence the book doesn't even mention anything about your baby and what she must eat or avoid. It just talks about you, what must you eat and specifically avoid. The book aims to put you in the best shape of your life, for the most stressful yet joyful job of being a mom. A full-time mom, a permanent mom, a mom for many lifetimes.

Though Kareena is the inspiration, the reason for this book is Taimur. He came along and disrupted my plans of writing a book for kids. Well, like a good aunt, I am only glad and grateful. Had it not been for him, a special book on pregnancy would have never happened. As I finish this book, I will get back on track to complete my book for kids. One that aims to nourish them, sets them free from wrong ideas about food and hopefully leaves them and their children in a world better than the one we brought them into.

With this in my heart, I hope you have enjoyed this book, found it useful, and will see you soon with the children's book. So long, yummy mommy!

Rujuta Diwekar
Mumbai
April 2017